treat your own frozen shoulder

a self-help guide using the
Niel-Asher technique™

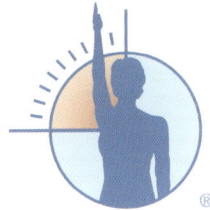

Simeon Niel-Asher ©

4th Edition 3rd reprint

acknowledgements

This book is dedicated to Galina, my parents and little Gypsy.
I would like to acknowledge the following people for their help, advice and support:

Roger and Susi Camrass, friends and advisors
Mr. Jonathan Middleburgh, Barrister
Anne Sweatbaum, PR
Alice Hart-Davis, Journalist
Michael Anderson & Jonathan Perham, Coutts & Co.
Marianne Vizincey-Lambert Sarah Weldon Karina Spero and Julia Spicer Osteopaths
Decherts Law firm, S.J. Berwin
Tony Orsi
Geoff Catini & the team at www.netro42.com
Especially to all of my wonderful patients

warning

This treatment has proven safe and easy to use. However, the following warning has been placed on this guide.

disclaimer

This book is not intended as a substitute for medical advice. The reader should regularly consult a physician or health care professional in matters relating to health and particularly in respect of any symptoms which may require diagnosis or medical attention. In the majority of cases of frozen shoulder syndrome there is no underlying illness or cause. However a proper diagnosis from a registered practitioner is advised. If you perform this treatment it is at your own risk.

the Niel-Asher technique™ is a registered trademark

The Niel-Asher technique™ Patent pending

A list of practitioners of the Niel-Asher technique and their locations can be found on the website **www.frozenshoulder.com** which is regularly updated. Because this technique is new there may not be a practitioner near you. Please bear with us; we are endeavouring to teach The Niel-Asher technique™ worldwide. A list of courses and dates is also available on the website, so please inform your practitioner.

NB: The Niel-Asher technique™ is taught only to practitioners with an existing medical or physical therapy qualification who belong to a recognised Register. Only practitioners who have been on an accredited course are recognised, so please check the website.

Editor, Jonathan Brodkin, Joanna Baruch

Art direction, Greg Jakobek   Design, Dom Cooper and Simon Mok at Warsaw
Photography, Ian Jackson   Ali G photograph, © 2002 David Scheinmann
Models, Kathy Hill and Billy Waters
Illustration, Sarah Pike
Towels supplied courtesy of Jasper Conran

Printed by Creative Production Ltd.
This book is printed on paper from sustainable forests.

contents

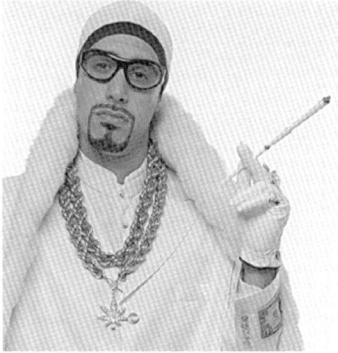

Ali G *icon/superstar*

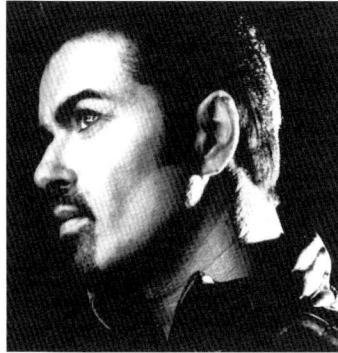

Yo Simeon,
muff respek
2da macdaddy d
shoulders
ALIG

George Michael *singer/songwriter*

'I am delighted to recommend Simeon as an osteopath. His work with me has always been excellent. He is a great bloke and I hope you all gain benefit from his new technique for treating your frozen shoulders.'

Martin Kemp *actor*

'I first encountered Simeon's work in 1998 when he helped to heal me after surgery for my two brain tumours. Simeon's was the strongest, most powerful form of treatment I have ever experienced. I highly recommend him and his work and wish him luck with his pioneering work with frozen shoulder syndrome.'

Victoria Wood *comedienne*

'As a very satisfied patient of Simeon's, I am happy to recommend his work to a wider public and wish him well with his revolutionary new treatment for frozen shoulders.'

foreword

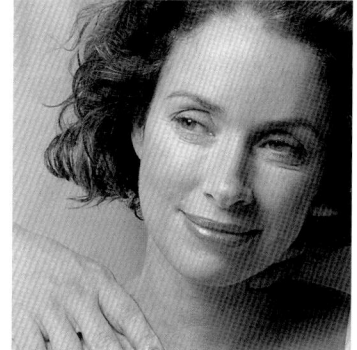

I first saw Simeon in March 2000 with a right sided 'classic frozen shoulder' at least, that is what the surgeon told me. I was in constant pain and couldn't sleep; it was as if my life was plagued. As a professional model I was using my arms all the time and had to smile for the camera, even though I often wanted to wince.

My problem had been on going for over a year before I saw Simeon. The pain had gradually worsened and then became unbearable. I had been to my GP who had given me two steroid injections; which didn't help. I had seen a physiotherapist about 30 times and had seen two other Osteopaths and a manipulative physical therapist; all to no avail. I was desperate and when the surgeon told me he wanted to manipulate my shoulder under anaesthetic I was scared. I typed in 'frozen shoulder' on the web and to my great luck Simeon's excellent website appeared. It was full of helpful advice and I immediately booked to see him. Within three sessions my pain had disappeared. On the fourth session I was totally cured.

Simeon,

I cannot begin to express my gratitude; I thought my career was over. I wish you the best of luck with your book. I recommend your treatment to everyone and hope they get results as good as mine.

It therefore gives me great pleasure to be your model for this book - as a real patient who has successfully been cured with your unique treatment method.

Yours truly,

Kathy Hill

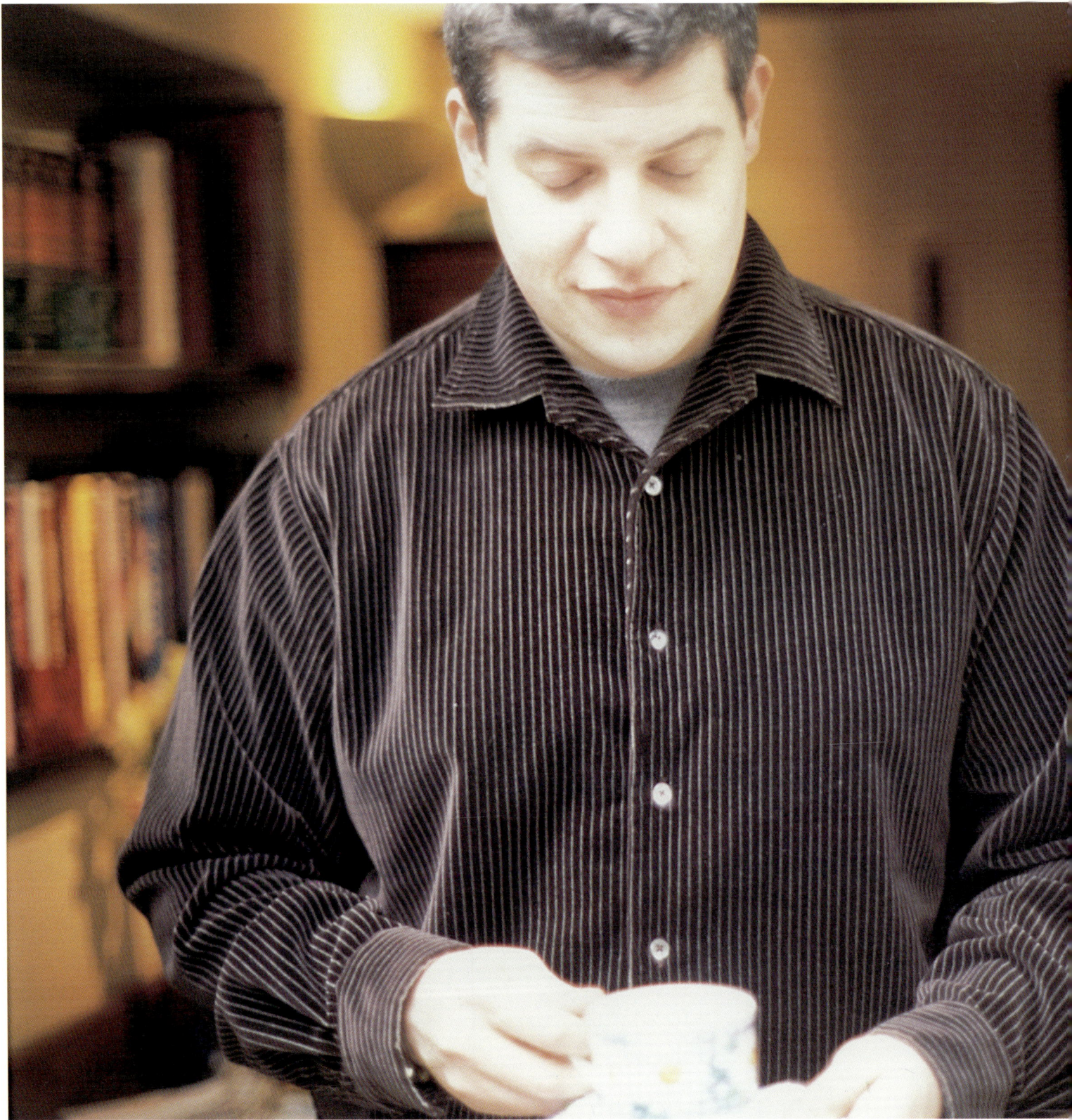

welcome

Welcome to my self-help guide. The technique that I have invented is hands on. It will require a partner or therapist to get the best results. I have written this guide due to the overwhelming demand for information about my treatment. As you will see, it is a straightforward technique. It does, however, require some skill and sensitivity on the part of the person performing it but I maintain that as long as the patient is treated with love and respect anyone can have success with my method.

This guide is aimed mainly at the treatment of frozen shoulder syndrome. This is probably the most difficult shoulder condition that occurs. It is often the end point of many other types of shoulder complaint. Because a frozen shoulder affects almost every tissue of the shoulder joint, my technique has proven successful with many other short, and long-standing shoulder problems.

I would always advise any prospective patient to seek a diagnostic opinion from a qualified medical practitioner before using my method. As we will see, several conditions can mimic a frozen shoulder and some of them may require more serious medical attention. This guide, then, is aimed at the person who has seen a medical doctor or physical therapist and has been diagnosed as having a 'frozen shoulder'. You may have been through several months of symptoms and I know many of you will be in a great deal of pain. The technique has proven effective at any stage of a frozen shoulder, but due to the massive amount of swelling in the first three months, it seems to work best after four to six months of symptoms. In my own clinic I usually treat a patient once per week/ten days for six or seven sessions. However, I would recommend you or your partner perform it every fourth day, gently, for four to ten weeks. I have also found that the longer the symptoms have been there, the quicker and easier the treatment. For example, someone who comes to me with a frozen shoulder of eighteen months duration usually responds to about four sessions. This might sound strange but I will explain my theory later.

For the best results I would recommend reading the book once or twice before attempting to perform the technique. I have tried to make it a simple and accessible text. I have used photographs of me and my colleagues to break up and personalise the text. Any medical words that you are not familiar with are translated at the back of the guide. For more information, please look at the website www.frozenshoulder.com

It is my sincere hope that you find this guide useful and every one of you gets some benefit from it. It is quite difficult to teach through a book a technique that has taken six years to develop. Some of it relies on a type of tissue sensitivity that comes with practice. If you follow the guide carefully I am sure you will succeed. I wish you all success and pray that my method brings you relief.

Simeon

the bare bones of the matter

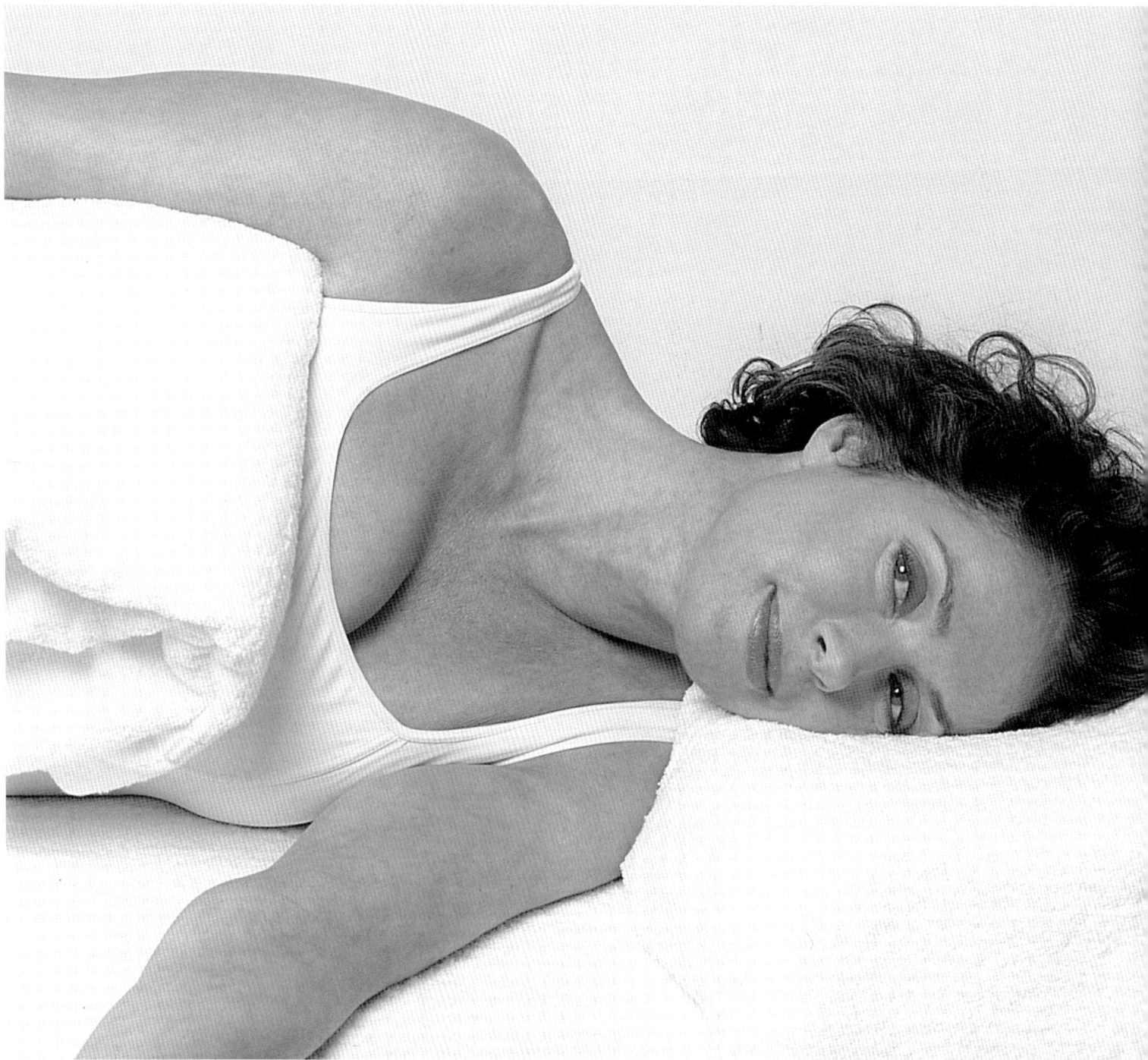

shoulder anatomy

The shoulder is one of the most complicated joints in the body. This is because it is really a series of four joints that work together with co-ordinated precision. The easiest way to understand the shoulder is to break it down into its constituent parts; then we can assemble it and try to make sense of it with reference to your living shoulder.

After looking at the living anatomy of the shoulder we will move away from the muscles and bones and look more towards patterns of movement.

overview

Understanding what the shoulder looks like below the skin will give us clues as to the causes of shoulder pain. We are going to concentrate on the bones and the ligaments; then we will look at some of the muscles that co-ordinate movement of the shoulder joint.

It is important to note that we are now looking at the ideal situation. Many factors affect the proper alignment of the shoulder joints such as:

- Posture
- Injury
- Occupation
- Ageing
- Sport
- Stress
- Illness
- Emotion

Because it is such a robust and adaptable system consisting of many joints, the shoulder compensates for these factors over the years. It makes minute adjustments in each of its components. Unfortunately, a time comes when it can no longer compensate for these factors; this is often when pain sets in. Because a frozen shoulder usually asserts itself between the ages of 40 and 70 it is more than likely that a combination of all the above factors will be implicated, as we will later explain.

bones

Man walks upright. That will come as no surprise, I am sure. The thing is that we are still co-ordinated (and neurologically wired) as if we walk on all fours. That is why when you walk (or march) you will naturally find a rhythm of swinging the opposite arms and legs, so it may help to think of the shoulder girdle as a modified front leg. The shoulder ball and socket (gleno-humeral) joint is highly specialised for performing its duties. It allows a vast range of movement, more than any other joint in the body. It acts both as a centre of movement and as a stabiliser for elbow, wrist and hand movements. The ability to manipulate objects with our hands is perhaps the single most important difference between humans and other animals. And we do this in just about every aspect of our daily life. Yet there is a price to pay for this massive amount of shoulder 'mobility', namely a decrease in shoulder 'stability'. Compare this to the hip joint, which is very stable (hardly ever dislocating) but does not have a large amount of mobility. So the shoulder relies heavily on its bones, ligaments and muscles for strength, stability and function.

Its only bony attachment to the body is by a short thin strut called the collar-bone (clavicle). The rest of the shoulder girdle is held in alignment by a co-ordinated series of muscular contractions.

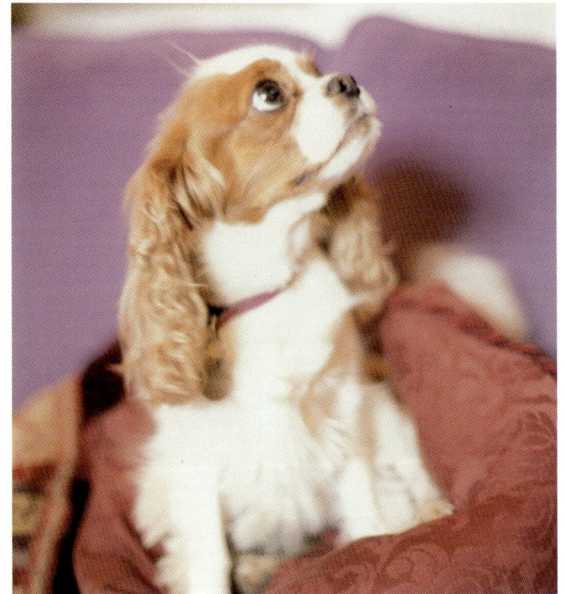

Gypsy dreams about bones!

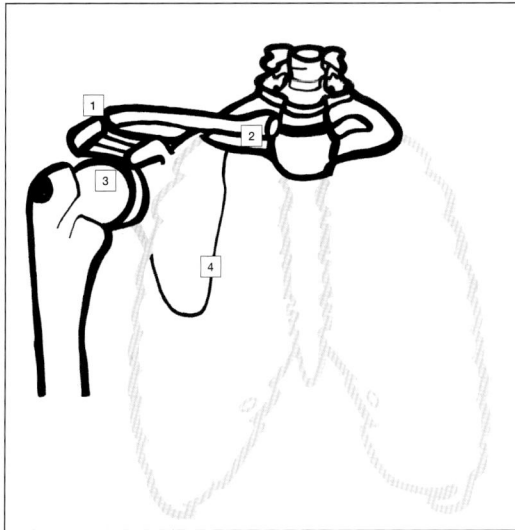

1 Acromio-clavicular joint

2 Sterno-clavicular joint

3 Gleno-humeral joint

4 Scapulo-thoracic joint

The shoulder consists of the upper arm bone (the humerus) and its connection to a cup on the shoulder blade (scapula), which is called the gleno-humeral joint. The secondary components are also important to note because, as described above, small adjustments are made here to compensate for changes during shoulder activities and posture. The secondary components are the collar-bone (clavicle) attaching to the breast-bone (sterno-clavicular joint) and shoulder blade (acromio-clavicular joint). And the muscular sliding joint of the shoulder blade and the back muscles (scapulo-thoracic joint).

This anatomy gives us landmarks that we can feel under the skin. Where the bones join each other is usually quite sensitive. It is probably worth taking a break at this point to practise feeling the joints. This will orientate you for the techniques described later.

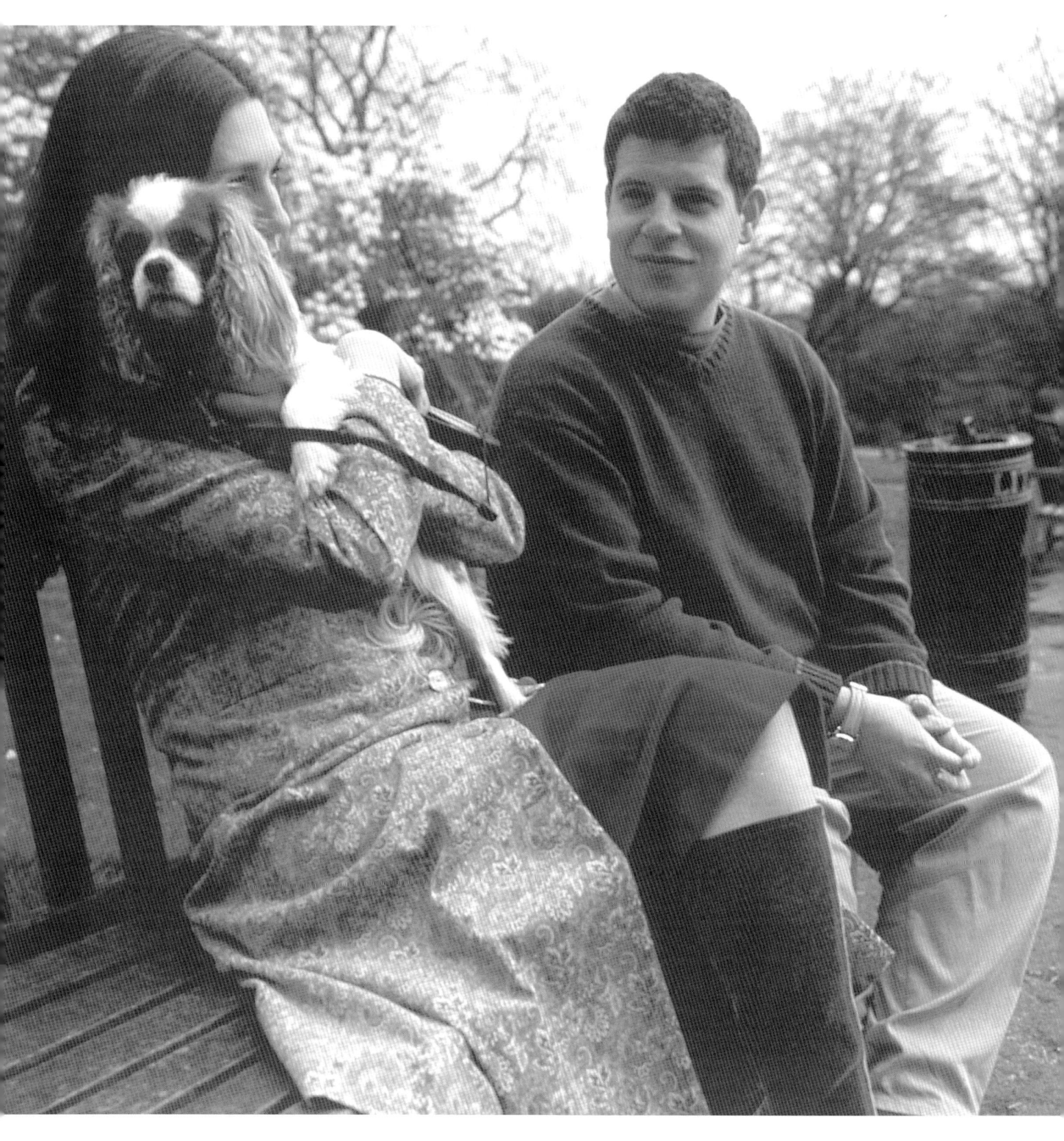

ligaments and the capsule

Because the shoulder girdle is so tenuously held in place, extremely tough and robust ligaments brace it. Current research has highlighted the role between the capsule (see later) and ligaments of the gleno-humeral joint as the origin of shoulder pain.

The vast majority of joints in the body are called synovial joints and they share a common format (or morphology). The gleno-humeral joint (ball and socket joint) is a synovial joint.

A dense tough substance called cartilage covers the bony surfaces where they meet each other. Surrounding the joint and its ligaments is the bag-like capsule, which contains the synovial fluid.

There are two aspects to the capsule. One is the synovial membrane, the other the capsular ligaments. The purpose of the synovial membrane is to lubricate the joint. It stops muscles and bones from rubbing directly on one another, and is filled with synovial fluid. The ligaments literally strap the joint. The membrane is covered on its outside wall by the capsule. At certain places on its exterior the capsule thickens and condenses into ligamentous bands (see diagram).

This bag is somewhat different in the shoulder to other joints. As you can see in the diagrams it spreads quite far around the shoulder joint. It 'intercommunicates' with other synovial membranes that cover other bones and muscles of the shoulder joint and, notably, it covers one of the biceps tendons as it makes its journey to the ball and socket.

The amount of synovial fluid contained in a healthy shoulder joint is about 30-40ml (this is a large amount when compared to other joints). It is interesting to note that some surgical studies have demonstrated that there is as little as 5ml in a frozen shoulder. The fluid itself is slightly viscous; it is produced from specialised cells that line the membrane and the joint and is squeezed out by the normal motion of the joint. This lubricating fluid also nourishes the cartilage of the joint, especially when damaged. This compounds the problem of a frozen shoulder where the tiny amount of fluid leaves the joint dry inside, further straining the innate repair mechanisms.

The injured biceps tendon may also be a major factor in all shoulder pain syndromes. It originates deep in the ball and socket joint and runs right through the synovial membrane. Any inflammation can spread quickly and directly from the inflamed biceps tendon into the ball and socket joint itself.

The inflammation makes the viscous synovial fluid thicker and stickier, like glue. As you can imagine, this greatly hinders normal joint functioning.

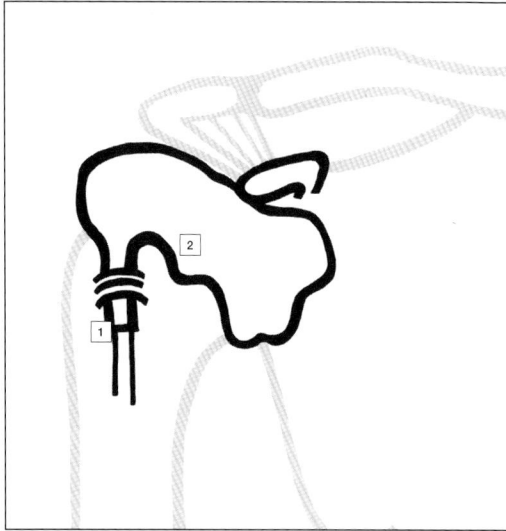

1 Biceps tendon and tendon's sheath
2 Capsular bag

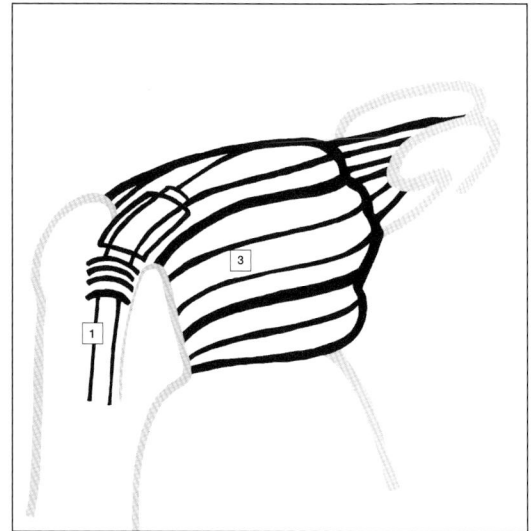

1 Biceps tendon and tendon's sheath
3 Capsular fibres

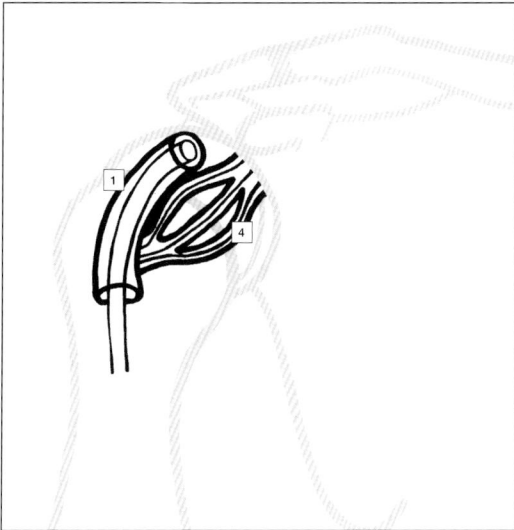

1 Biceps tendon and tendon's sheath
4 Thickenings / ligamentous bands

These bands have several functions. Mainly they serve to stabilise the joint in certain planes of movement, preventing dislocation. Current research has indicated that these bands or ligaments may play a crucial role in shoulder pain, especially in the development of a 'frozen shoulder'. It has recently been demonstrated that shortening (ageing and repeated damage) of the front / bottom (anterior-inferior) capsular ligament is a primary cause of frozen shoulder syndrome.

movement

As discussed earlier, the shoulder joints allow a vast range of movement, more than any other joint in the body. To simplify things we will talk only about the 'pure' movements of flexion, extension, abduction, adduction, and internal and external rotation (see below). In reality, however, all movements we make are made up of infinite combinations of these pure movements.

Problems with the neck, elbow, wrist and hand will also be affected by the way we use our shoulders.

We shall therefore divide movement into various planes:

Flexion is the straight forward/front movement (it has a range of up to 180°).

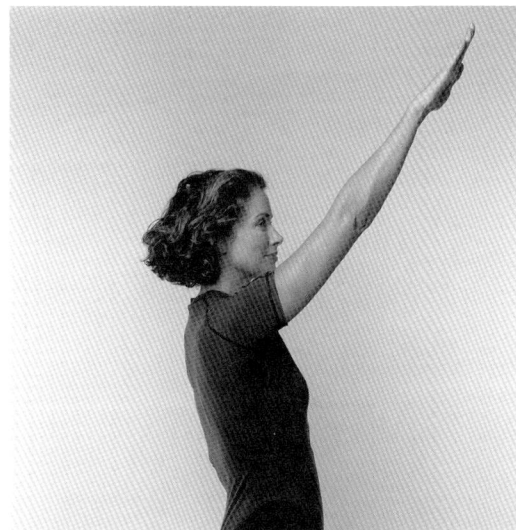

Flexion

Extension is the straight backward movement (it has a range of 70°).

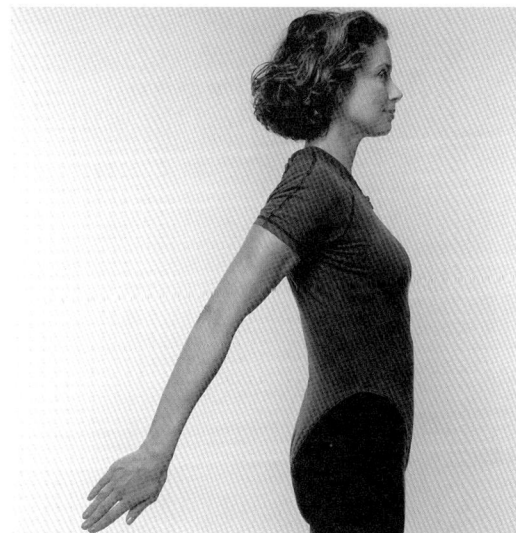

Extension

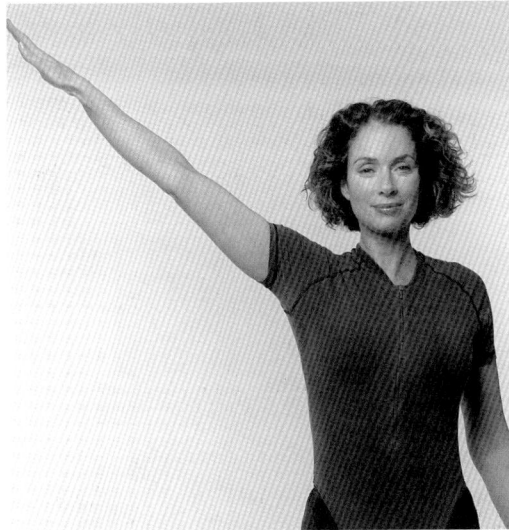

Abduction

Abduction is the sideways movement away from the body (it has a range of 180°).

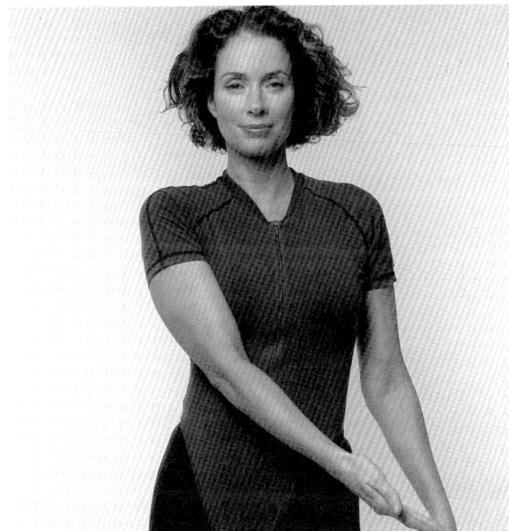

Adduction

Adduction is the sideways movement towards the body (it has a range of 30°).

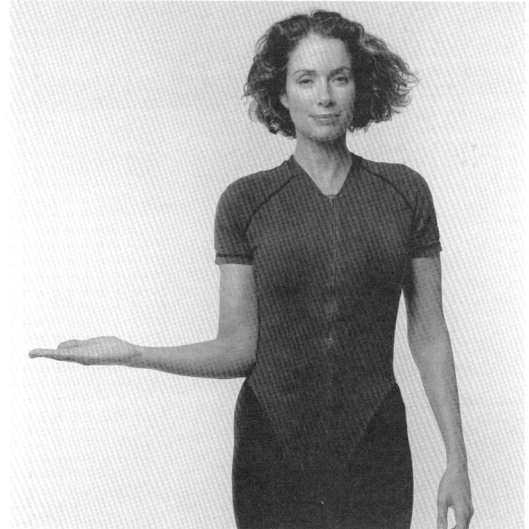

External rotation

External rotation means turning the hand outward with the elbow tucked tight into the side and the elbow bent so the arm is straight (it has a range of 80°).

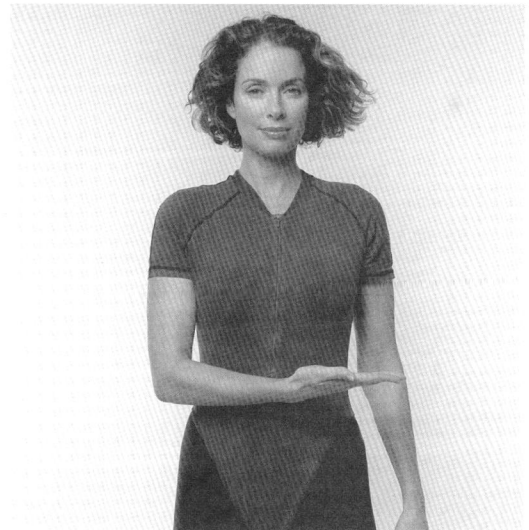

Internal rotation

Internal rotation means turning the hand inward (it has a range of 95°).

In reality, movements are 'complex' which means they are composed of many combined patterns. Putting your hand into your back pocket, for example, involves extension, adduction and internal rotation. It also involves a slight compensatory twist of the spine and pelvis involving many sets of muscles.

muscles

As stated previously the muscles of the shoulder have a dual role. They support and maintain the shoulder posture, and they also move the arm and shoulder into position as required. It is important to discuss some of these muscles as they may be directly related to your shoulder pain. The way the body repairs muscle damage is also of direct relevance for many shoulder complaints.Unfortunately, anatomists have chosen Latin names for these muscles. They describe features of the muscle (i.e. biceps means two heads) but they can be difficult to understand at first. I will do my best to simplify things where possible.

Two main groups of muscles stabilise the shoulder. One is collectively known as the rotator cuff and the other as the deltoid muscle. They collectively help to pull the ball into the socket and they also serve to move the shoulder in various directions. The rotator cuff is a muscular cuff made up of several muscles: mainly the supraspinatus muscle, then the infraspinatus, the teres minor and the subscapularis muscle. These muscles blend together as they connect to the arm bone (humerus) with a common tendon (called the conjoint tendon); this is an area of potential vulnerability and is a common source of shoulder pain.

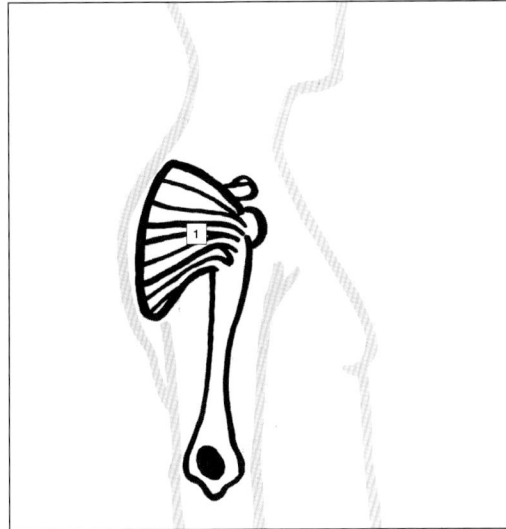

1 Rotator cuff

Lying above the shoulder in a kind of dome is the powerful deltoid muscle. It has three components, each specialising in a certain direction of movement. The portion at the front (anterior) helps flexion, the back part (posterior) helps extension and the middle fibres give about 85% of the power for abduction (the other 15% comes from the supraspinatus muscle). The deltoid muscle lies just beneath the skin of the shoulder and connects to the bone about four inches down the outside of the arm. This is an area that is often lumpy to the touch in a frozen shoulder. It is one of the main areas that my treatment programme addresses.

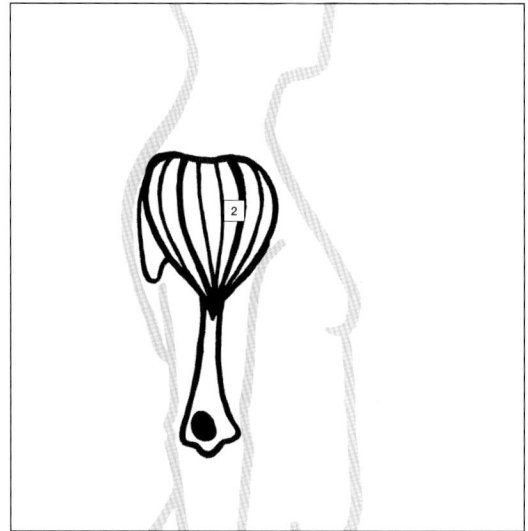

2 Deltoid muscle

the back

Other muscles that stabilise and move the shoulder joint are:

1 Trapezius

2 Levator scapulae

3 Rhomboids

4 Triceps

5 Latissimus dorsi

the front

1 Pectoral muscles

2 Subclavius muscles

3 Biceps

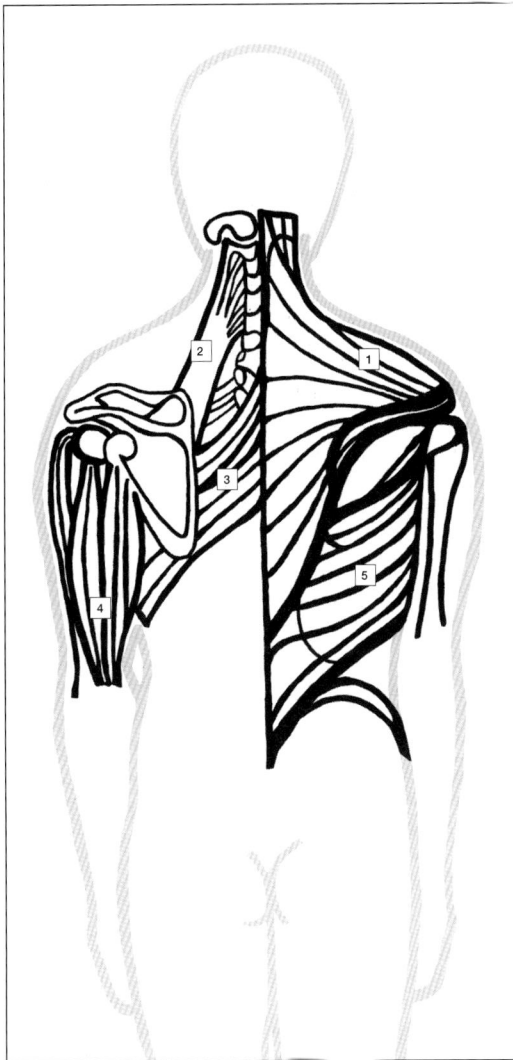
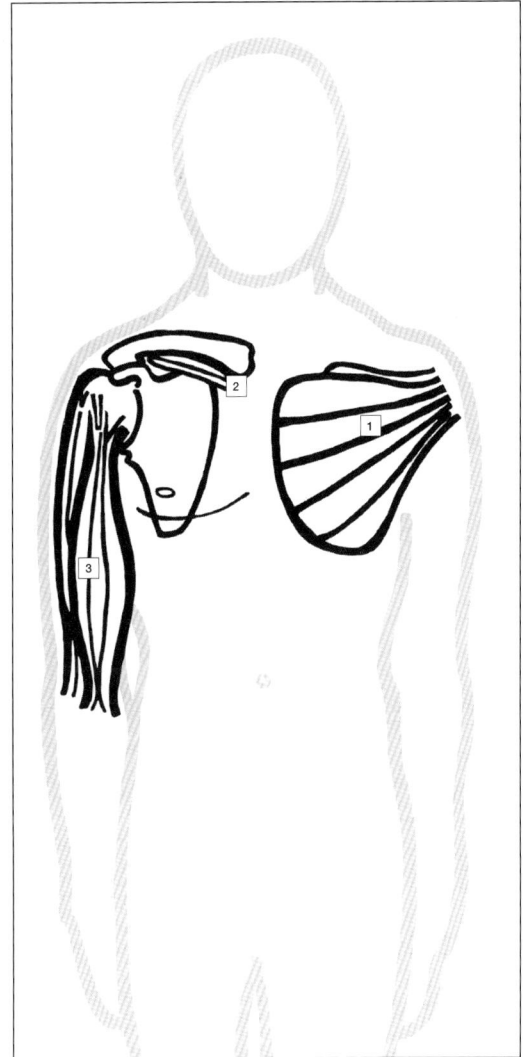

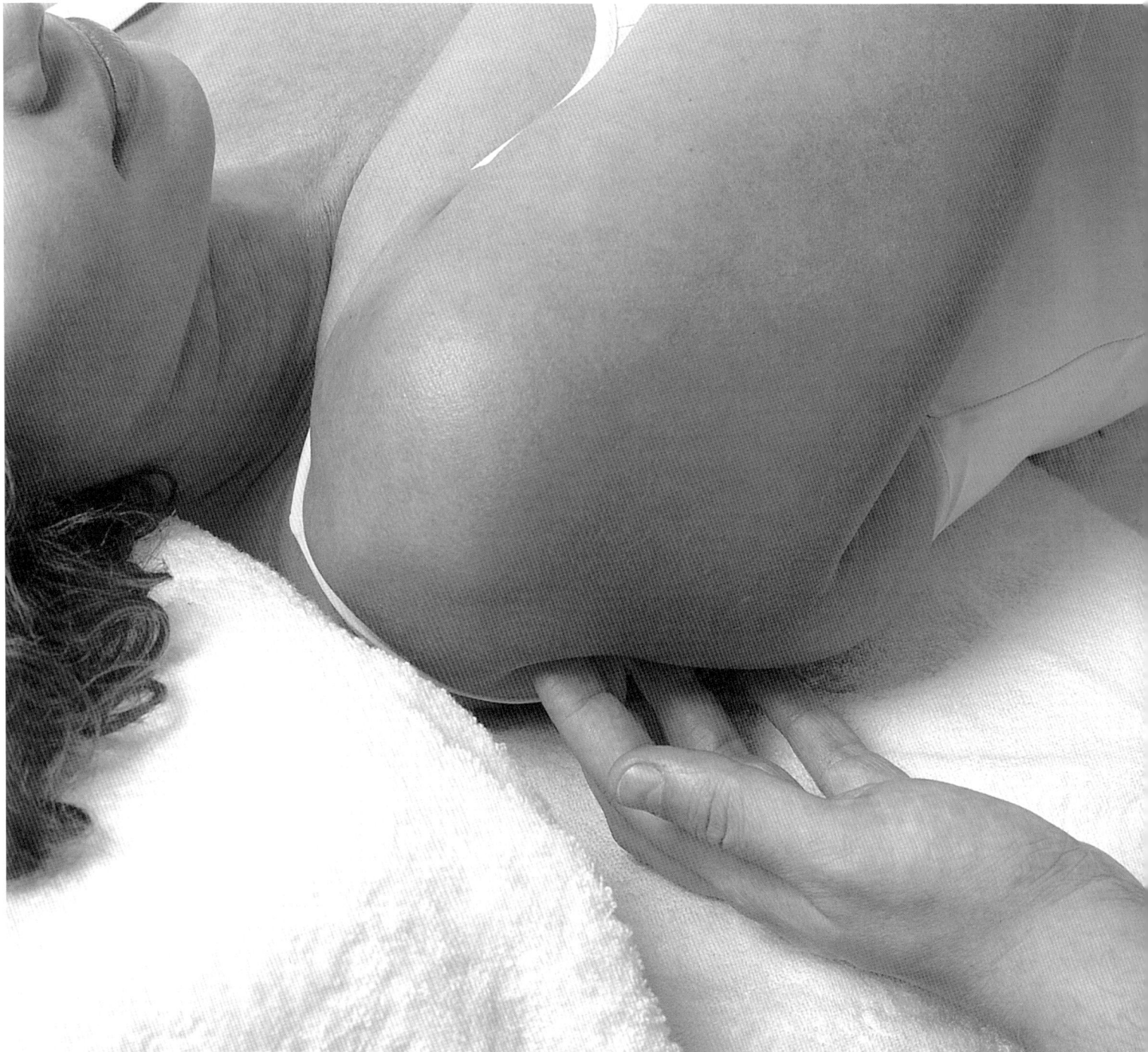

all about shoulder pain

After studying this chapter, you should be able to:

- Identify medical conditions that can cause shoulder pain
- Understand the mechanisms of shoulder injury
- Understand the theory behind the Niel-Asher Technique™

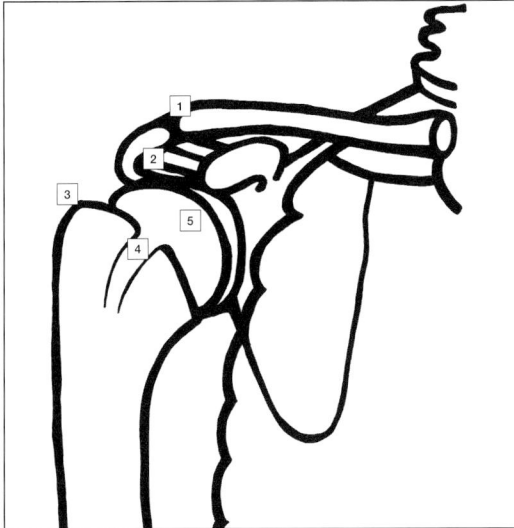

sites of shoulder pain

1 Acromio-clavicular joint

2 Sub-acromial bursa

3 Supraspinatus tendon insertion (rotator cuff)

4 Biceps tendon (long head)

5 Gleno-humeral joint

muscle wasting

Muscle wasting is a common feature of shoulder injury. This is either from a lack of use (such as a long-standing frozen shoulder) or from a change in the nerve supply to the muscles. Wasting appears as hollow areas or depressions around the shoulder. It can also be indicated when the shoulder blade is not suspended properly and seems to stick out (this is due to the wasting of the subscapularis muscle). If wasting is due to lack of use, then once the shoulder is moving fully, the wasted muscles tend to build up again within two-three months. If wasting is secondary to neurological damage, it is important to establish which nerves have been damaged and why. Again, please consult your doctor if you are worried.

Many patients with a frozen shoulder have reported to me that their muscle power and mass have rapidly wasted away, often within days of the shoulder becoming stiff. It may be interesting to note that after a fracture, muscle wasting occurs rapidly, literally within a few hours. This is obviously not due to lack of use. Studies have demonstrated that this wasting is a type of protective mechanism, which forces the injured area to rest; this may well be the case with a frozen shoulder as well.

wear, tear and repair — night pain

During the daytime, the weight of the arm itself cuts off some of the blood supply to the shoulder muscles. This is generally not problematic. However, when shoulder muscles are injured or damaged this has several important implications.

First, any muscle damage is not repaired during the daytime. This is because muscle damage needs a healthy blood supply to bring reparative cells and products to the damaged tissue and to remove toxins and worn cells from the damage site.

Secondly, this means that repair can only occur at night. When we lay down to sleep, there is no pull of gravity on the shoulder and the blood supply can flow freely. Most shoulder problems are worse at night because of the increased blood flow to tissues. These become readily swollen; the swelling pushes on other tissues and stimulates pain from small nerve endings. The swelling also attracts reparative cells which trigger inflammation.

In the case of frozen shoulder syndrome this night pain is doubled; partly because of the increased blood supply (in an attempt to repair) and partly because of the nature of inflammation. Inflammation is sticky. It draws water to the damaged area, and hence causes swelling. This swelling is worse at night as the arm is not being moved. Once the arm and shoulder are moved, the inflammatory swelling is dissipated, making the pain diminish. This is why, generally, the shoulder feels better during the daytime when the arm is being gently moved and much worse at night.

Often not all of the damage can be repaired in one night, and the next day the arm is used again with a certain amount of damage remaining within the shoulder muscles. If this process goes on for several weeks, a curious situation occurs. What seems to happen is that certain areas inside the damaged muscles (known as the critical zones) accumulate calcium molecules (chalk). This chalk is viewed as an irritant to the already damaged tissues and its presence triggers further bouts of inflammation which trigger further cycles of pain. The chalk also accumulates if there is enough, it can weaken the damaged muscle so much that it tears further. As you can see, this process can become a vicious circle.

the theory behind the practice

Over the years, I have come to realise that, in some ways, far from being complicated, the shoulder has a sublime simplicity to it. Reducing the shoulder down to muscles and bones is useful for understanding the structures but does not really give an understanding of the shoulder.

Movement is everything; I will use an analogy to explain what I mean. The muscles and joints are there to express movement. In a sense, the muscles and bones can be visualised as colours on an artist's palette. We all use them in subtle and different combinations for performing our daily activities. In this analogy, the brain is both an ever-changing three-dimensional canvas and the paint brush.

The key to understanding my unique approach to the shoulder requires us to examine the way the brain operates. The parts of the brain in which we are interested are those that control sensation and movement. We call these the sensory and motor cortex, which lies near the median fissure (central groove) of the cerebral hemispheres (see diagram).

We are born with a blueprint of the body 'hard-wired'

into our brain in the motor cortex. Here, all the co-ordinated instructions to the muscles take place. This is the control centre from where movement emanates via motor nerves. The motor cortex sends messages to the muscles and bones telling them how and where to move. These movements are learnt as we re-perform them. No muscle is moved 100% on its own. In reality, movement occurs in patterns (a combination of many muscles and joints, some remote). The brain remembers and stores these patterns of movement; it does not see the body in the reductionist way that we tend to.

But the motor cortex is only half the picture. The other half is the sensory cortex. It receives a constant stream of feedback from every muscle, joint and fibre of the body via sensory nerves. In fact, all our tissues are continually painting a picture to our brain. The brain is then able to constantly monitor our position in the space around us.

Our muscles, joints and connective tissues are perfused with a variety of sensory organs that give us feedback and connection to our physical world. These include temperature, pain, touch, length of muscle fibres and joint orientation. Every muscle in our body has a different mixture of sensors embedded in it. For example, the Latissimus dorsi (Lats) muscle shown on page 22 contains a mass of sensors to do with incremental wing-like movements. The Lats, as they are known, are in fact the wing muscles in birds. In humans they also operate as a modified type of wing muscle, giving the brain information about the position of the shoulders in space, as well as moving the shoulder blade.

Each muscle and joint therefore has a dual purpose. One is to receive commands for movement from the brain, and the other is to give information and feedback to the brain. Thus each forms a beautiful and mutually balanced system. The motor map with which we are born is a complete map in itself, but it relies on feedback from the sensory map to re-enforce its image of itself.

This is quite a profound thought so let me explain it by an example. Until recently, the condition called phantom limb pain was something of a mystery to medicine.

This occurs in a small percentage of people who have been born without a limb, or who have lost a limb due to an accident or surgery. These people say that they can feel pain in the limb that is missing. They often describe the pain as 'a constant twisted pain', as if the limb has been 'shrunk' and is 'gnarled'. It can keep some people awake all night and is truly a miserable condition. It is made worse by the fact there is no limb to treat and therefore nowhere to put an anaesthetic; and often it does not even respond to painkillers. Recent studies have demonstrated that this condition may result from a lack of communication between the sensory and motor maps. At birth, there is a full four-limbed map of the body hard wired into the motor cortex. However, when the limb has gone, there is no sensory feedback mechanism to re-enforce the motor map. The brain gets confused and this, it has been suggested, may lead to phantom pain, where the brain invents pain as a result of this lack of referencing.

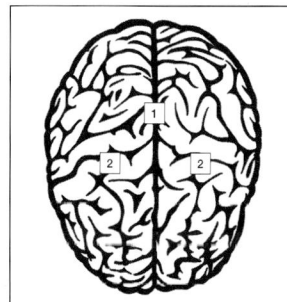

1 The median fissure
2 Sensory and motor cortex

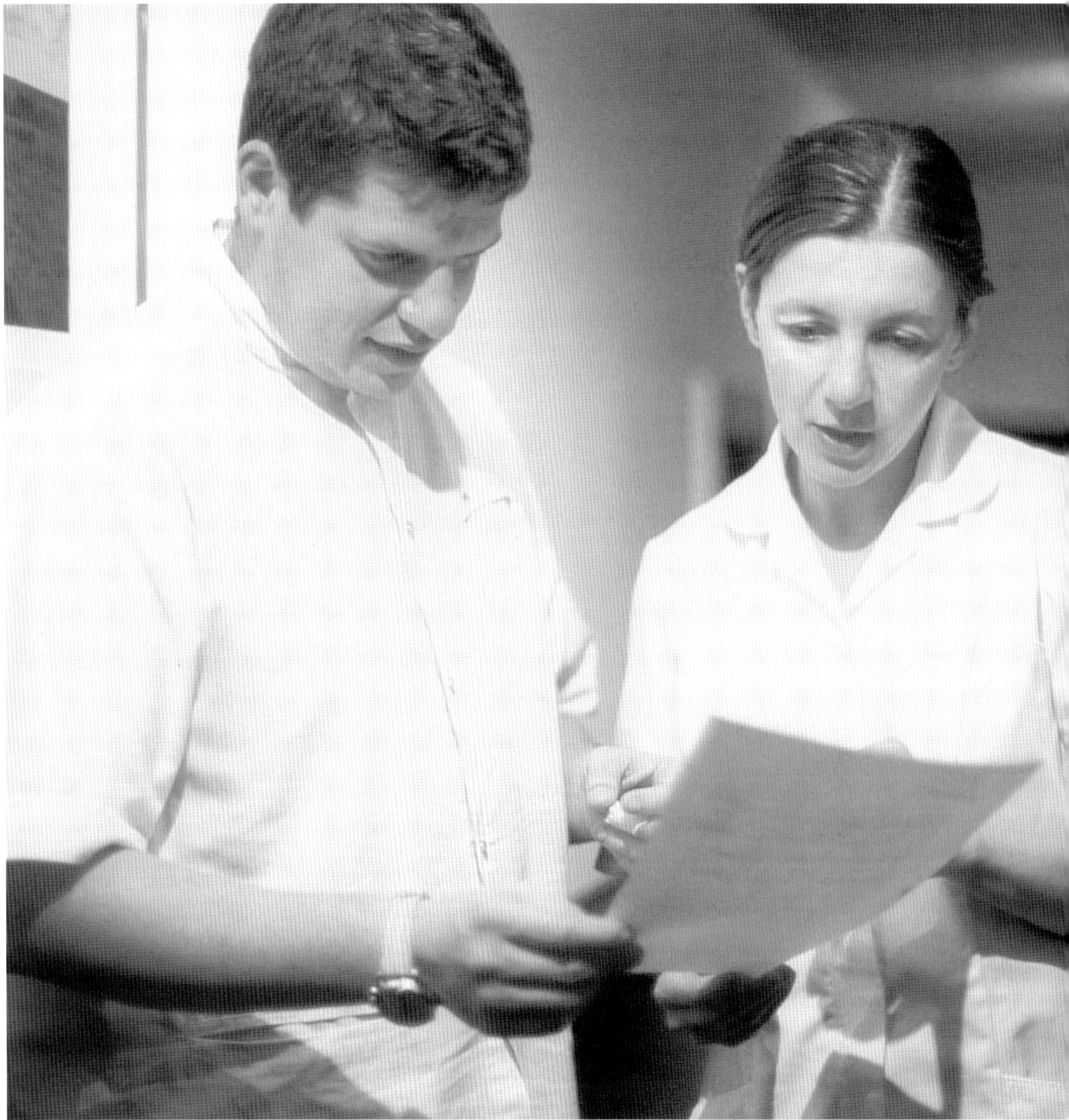

rules and patterns of movement

We can now think in terms of evolutionary patterns of movement. The brain seeks to translate our desire to, say, pick up a cup, into a movement pattern. To do this, it works thousands of fibres in dozens of muscles in a co-ordinated manner. To make it easier to control muscles, certain rules have had to be followed.

rule 1
direction and velocity of movement

There are only three types of movement that any living organism is capable of. These are forward/backward (flexion/extension), side to side (side bending) and rotation. In evolutionary terms, these basic types of movement have been combined over the millennia. Humans are able to perform three types of movement, whereas, for example, a primitive flatworm has only two of these movement patterns. Muscle groups and fibres have become specialised to express these three movement patterns. They are fundamentally different and require specialised co-ordination to mix all three together. A combination of all three planes of movement affords us the full range of mobility that we use for everyday tasks.

Different areas of the body are more specialised for different movement patterns. The shoulder joint has the most available movement patterns of any body joint. It is very mobile at the expense of stability. Shoulder dislocations, especially forwards, backwards or upwards, are fairly common.

rule 2
co-ordination

An important part of how my technique works can be understood in the context of co-ordinated muscle activity. We now know that the brain co-ordinates muscles in patterns as a result of the motor hardwiring.

No muscle works alone: when we move any muscle there is an in-built pattern of reciprocal muscle tension that is triggered. The brain has a programmed set of patterns in response to the changes in spatial position which movement causes. These compensatory responses adjust muscles and joints all over the body, from head to toe. The way the body is wired is in patterns. When a muscle is used (prime mover), it has an equal and opposite partner (antagonist), which is under reciprocal tension.

Movement is initiated by a desire to move (e.g. the desire to put on a coat). This desire is then translated by the brain into an energy-efficient way of carrying out the activity. The biological constraints of movement dictate that the body will always try to triangulate forces wherever it can: one point, e.g. the shoulder blade, is fixed still (by fixators), another is being moved in one direction, e.g. bending the arm (by a prime mover), while an equal and opposite movement (by an antagonist) takes place.

triangulated movement

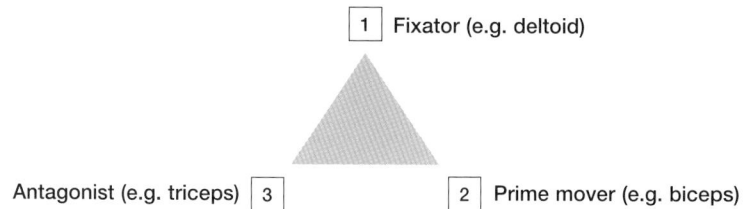

1 Fixator (e.g. deltoid)

Antagonist (e.g. triceps) 3

2 Prime mover (e.g. biceps)

This is the way that our motor cortex co-ordinates all movement. It may seem complicated at first but because it is the fundamental building block of all movements I would like to explore the process further.

Patterns of co-ordination can best be explained by looking at real-life examples.

the action of curling a weight using the biceps muscle

Here the weight trainer sits on a bench curling a dumbbell from the floor up to his or her shoulder, by bending the forearm in flexion. This is a simple model, but the principles behind it are common to most movement patterns.

In order for the weight to be lifted from the ground, the shoulder has to be kept stable and still; muscles called fixators do this. The muscle that curls up the arm is the biceps; in this example, the biceps acts as a prime mover. At the same time, the muscle at the back of the arm called the triceps is forced to relax; this muscle acts as an antagonist.

In this case, there is a direct neurological relationship between the biceps (prime mover) and triceps (antagonist). That is to say, if the biceps is 50% contracted, the triceps is 50% contracted. In order for the biceps to be 90% contracted, the triceps is automatically 10% contracted. This fixed pattern is, in my opinion, at the centre of frozen shoulder syndrome.

Curling the biceps on its own is a simple example of movement. Tasks such as washing the hair or doing up the bra are much more complex. Even so all patterns of movement have fixators, prime movers and antagonists. What happens in these cases is that all of the movements patterns required are superimposed and orchestrated effortlessly by the motor cortex. However, when one or more muscle is unable to function properly the whole system is forced to compromise and adapt.

If the shoulder joints have, for example, arthritis or the posture is 'round shouldered' the brain has to adapt by recruiting other muscle groups to achieve movement. Because we are all shaped differently and may have different ways of holding ourselves against gravity (posture), we vary slightly in the pattern of muscles used even for the same actions. I would use a slightly different combination of muscles in brushing my hair from you. In the normal course of things this does not matter a great deal, but it indicates that far from being a simple question of one muscle performing one task, the relationship of the motor cortex to our muscles is not fixed. It is in fact 'plastic', that is to say certain muscles are ideal for certain jobs but if they are damaged or injured the brain will find other ways to re-route power to other muscles.

In frozen shoulder syndrome, the brain is forced to re-organise all movement patterns due to the swelling and tethering of certain muscle sheaths. The brain is then forced to recruit different muscles as prime movers and antagonists. The body will strive to maintain movement for as long as possible but eventually, as the co-ordinationed relationships deteriorate, movement becomes rapidly limited. Furthermore, in my opinion, some sort of neurological switching takes place where the prime mover/antagonists relationship gets switched around.

The way the motor cortex changes its co-ordination pattern in frozen shoulder syndrome is the same for everyone. By observing the way in which it adapts, I have developed the key to 'defrosting' the frozen shoulder. And by using a choreographed series of co-ordinated pressure points, I have been able to find a way to fool the brain into switching the confused neurological and muscular relationships back to normal.

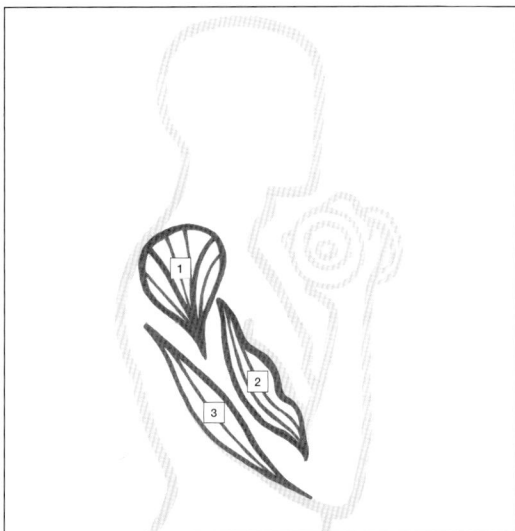

treatment topography

The treatment I have developed is hands on. It involves using a sequenced series of pressure points and stretching manoeuvres. Some of it can be painful while other parts are soothing. This is for a reason. As we have discussed, the tissues of the body have many types of receptors embedded within them. Some respond to deep touch, others to superficial touch, some to pain, others to hot or cold. All of our human experience of our environment is mediated through our tissues' sensory receptors. Our tissues sense the world around us and translate these sensations into messages that our brain decodes.

It has always been my belief that physical therapy should contain as many types of sensation as possible. This is so that the brain can get as much feedback about a damaged area as possible. In fact, I see treatment like a landscape. It should have mountains as well as valleys, peaks as well as troughs. Pain itself is an important feedback for the brain. All too often we avoid painful sensations. This is an in-built mechanism. However, gently reproducing the pain in a therapeutic situation can be extremely beneficial when combined with gentler and less painful stimuli.

Physical therapy often involves a sequence of manoeuvres. I think that it is not so much the manoeuvres that matter as the feedback profile that these manoeuvres create in the brain. Each manoeuvre stimulates a different profile (set of nerve impulses) depending which tissues and nerve endings are stimulated.

Another analogy that may help to understand the way my treatment works is that of a dialogue. The body and brain are in a constant state of dialogue. If you do not exercise or move around very much, the brain gets used to this diminished set of feedback mechanisms and adapts accordingly. If you are a walker or play sport, the feedback from the muscles to the brain during these activities creates a pattern, a type of vocabulary for the nervous system. The less activity you do the less rich the vocabulary. In the case of a frozen shoulder (as in many other physical complaints) the dialogue has become greatly limited. The technique I have developed, if performed in the correct order, stimulates and re-awakens this vocabulary thus allowing the body and nervous system to communicate again. Similarly, in general, the more physical activity we do the greater the vocabulary to the brain and the greater the sense of self-awareness. I personally have found gentle yoga seems to create a tremendous amount of mind — body vocabulary.

My technique differs from other physical therapy techniques not so much by what is done, but by the order in which it is performed. It is like a recipe, which is why I have developed this theme throughout the book. It is the order in which it is performed that stimulates the damaged tissues to fire off different signals to the brain. These signals are in specific sequences. They re-establish the relationships between the sensory feedback and the motor map within the brain.

My technique uses the various types of sensory feedback from the injured shoulder muscles to re-programme the frozen shoulder and defrost it.

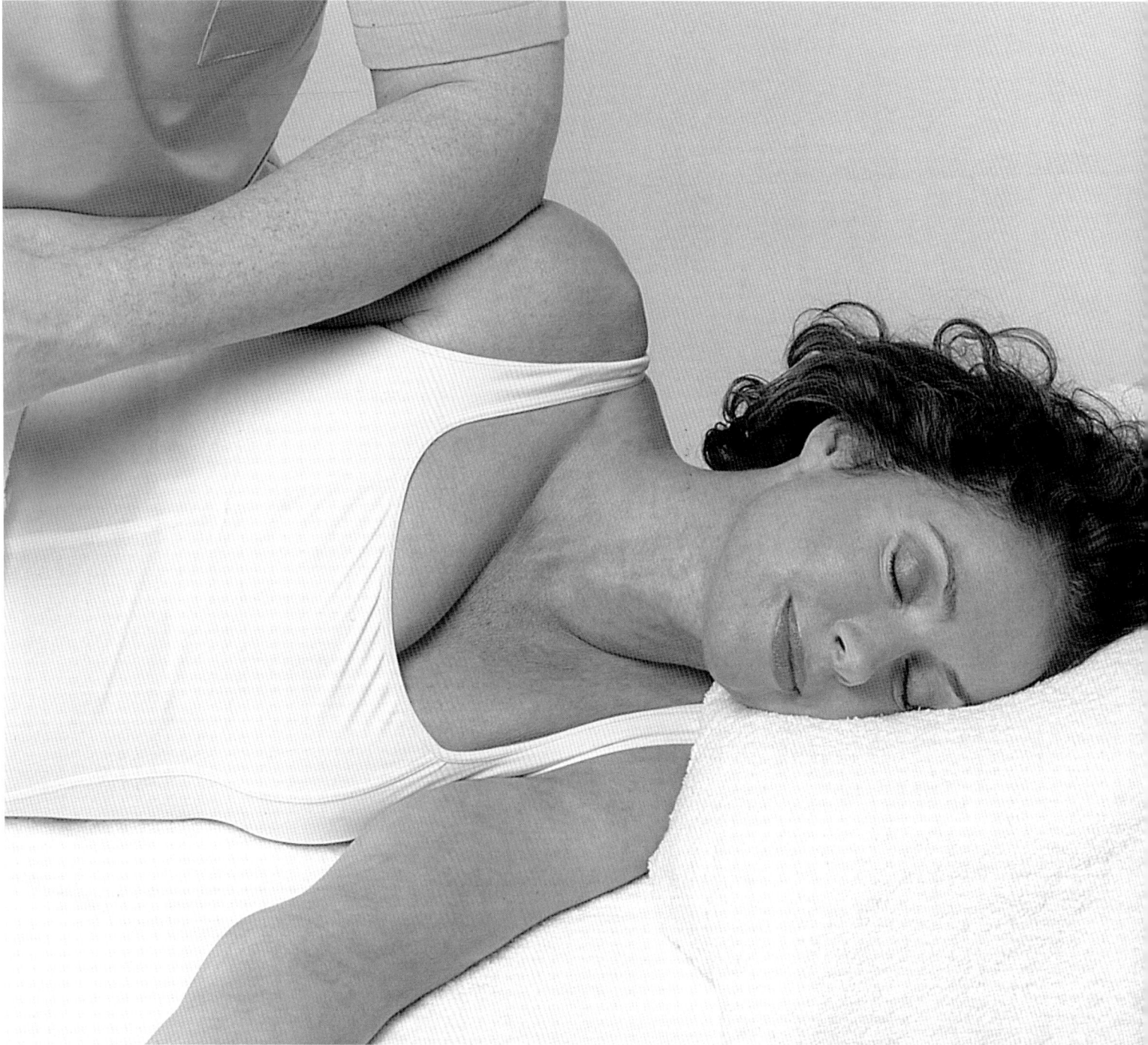

unravelling the frozen shoulder

frozen shoulder syndrome

Frozen shoulder syndrome is common, and affects 2-5% of the population. The French doctor ES Duplay first described it in 1872. Dr Duplay noticed that a group of patients seemed to present him with similar stories. He thought that the 'painful' and 'stiff' shoulders were the result of damage to the soft tissues (i.e. muscles) and not the joints; he termed the condition peri-arthritis. Since then many others have tried to define and explore the condition. The colloquial term 'frozen shoulder' was coined in 1934 by the American Dr E A Codman. It should be noted that some doctors use the term 'frozen shoulder' as a catch-all diagnosis for any shoulder pain. Other names include:

- Adhesive capsulitis
- Duplay syndrome
- Peri-arthritis of the shoulder
- 50's shoulder
- Irritative capsulitis
- Scapulo-humeral peri-arthritis
- Humero-scapular fibrositis
- Bursitis calcerea
- Stiff and painful shoulder
- The shoulder portion of shoulder–hand syndrome

As can be seen, even the name of the condition is the subject of medical debate. If authorities cannot agree on a name, a simple definition is even harder to find. This is because, until now, no one has found a consistent/reproducible technique or method for treating the condition. My hope is that over the next decade more and more doctors and therapists will come to practise and understand my radically different approach to this problem.

Most doctors' use the following definition, after NT Grubbs (physical therapist, Arkansas, USA) who defines frozen shoulder as 'a soft tissue capsular lesion accompanied by painful and restricted active and passive motion at the gleno-humeral joint'. The important point here is that the arm is stiff in both active and passive movement, i.e. neither patient nor doctor can lift the arm above a certain limited height.

incidence

Frozen shoulder affects slightly more females than males typically between 40 and 60 years of age. The non-dominant arm (i.e. left arm in most people) is more likely to be involved, although about 12% of people are affected on both sides (bilaterally). If both shoulders freeze, I have found that the second shoulder overlaps by about 6–9 months. Frozen shoulder syndrome is much more common in diabetics, affecting between 10 and 20%. We will discuss this later. It lasts for an average of 30 months, although one recently published study showed that up to 60% of people still had some symptoms after 10 years. All experts agree that, in the long term, it is preferable to have some sort of physical therapy, although some say that physical therapy is only of benefit after 12–18 months. It is worth pointing out that my method has been successful from three months onwards, and that the longer the symptoms have been there the quicker my method seems to work.

natural history

The natural history of this condition is well documented. Over the course of 30 months the frozen shoulder passes through three phases: freezing, frozen and thawing.

- The freezing (painful) phase lasts between three and eight months. Severe night pain is a common feature of this phase. People often complain that they are unable to sleep on the affected side. If they do manage to drift off, they are soon awoken in agony. People find they are arranging pillows to support the arm and that they must 'steal' sleep where they can. The pain itself can be quite horrendous. People usually describe three types of pain to me:

  1. A constant 'internal' dull burning
  2. Pain down the outside of the upper arm
  3. Severe sharp catching pain after certain innocuous movements lasting up to two minutes

Along with this there can often be rapid stiffening of the whole shoulder. People usually report pain when brushing the hair, doing up the bra or reaching behind them.

- This is followed by the frozen (stiff) phase, which lasts between four and 12 months. There may still be night pain but this usually diminishes as shoulder mobility decreases. Here patients are usually able to sleep but find it increasingly difficult to perform daily chores. This case is especially so for those poor people who are affected on both sides. So many of the menial tasks we thoughtlessly perform become titanic achievements. I have had several female patients who have taken to wearing wigs, as they are unable to do their hair. Pain can often radiate into the forearm or hand, and in some cases the hand can become swollen and painful.
This may be the result of a condition called reflex sympathetic dystrophy (RSD).
The pain may also start at the back of the shoulder in the region of the triceps muscle, due to a triceps tendonitis (see page 37).

- Spontaneous recovery of mobility (thawing) follows over the next four to 12 months although full recovery is commonly protracted. Occasionally people may awake after 18 months to find they are fully better, but in my experience this is rare. Without treatment, even after the thawing phase a restriction of mobility may often persist for several years.

It is worth noting that some experts talk of a 'pre-adhesive' stage, before the freezing phase. Here patients present with signs and symptoms of what is termed 'impingement syndrome'. This is where there is still movement but there is a catching in certain positions. The only signs that there is a frozen shoulder would be if a camera were placed within the joint (arthroscopy). This reveals some reddening of the synovial capsule and an increase in thickening of the capsule.

movement

The most commonly affected movements are turning the bent arm outwards (external rotation) and lifting the arm sideways to the body (abduction) of the gleno-humeral joint. People commonly complain of sharp pain when reaching for the back pocket, combing the hair, or doing up the bra. Another action which patients find difficult is putting on a jacket or coat. The arm does not swing when walking. At rest, the arm is often held in a slightly guarded position (adduction and internal rotation), and the shoulder blade (scapula) of the affected side is usually held in an antalgic posture (to avoid pain it is elevated, laterally rotated and abducted). Depending on the longevity of symptoms, the body may develop a compensatory mechanical adaptation. This often leads to tense neck and shoulders, especially on the affected side. Because people become so dependent on their 'good arm' this may lead to tensions even here. I have found that regular simple neck and shoulder massage can be most helpful for this.

current treatments

Until now, there has been no consensus on the 'proper' method of treatment for the frozen shoulder. Numerous therapeutic regimes have been advocated, but none have proved consistently successful.

- The first line of treatment is usually a course of oral analgesic drugs such as NSAIDs, with or without physical therapy. There are many such drugs available. They can, however, cause side effects such as stomach upsets or skin rashes. (Some experts believe physical therapy is of little or no use during the freezing or frozen phases but may help speed up recovery during the thawing phase.)

- The GP may initiate a course of hydrocortisone injections into the shoulder, but these are rarely useful on their own. Most patients find that these provide relief for about two or three weeks.

- Patients may have more than a dozen physical therapy sessions including ultrasound, mobilisation and exercise regimens. Often the therapist tries to increase the range of motion by forcing the shoulder and arm to their limits. This is in my opinion totally incorrect. I have found that this method, as well as being extremely painful, has the opposite effect to that desired, and causes the shoulder to freeze even further. It is also reported by physical therapists that improvements come in waves and plateaus, making it frustrating and difficult to treat.

- Transcutaneous electrical nerve stimulation (TENS) machines are also commonly used to alleviate night pain. TENS units do not treat the problem; they are purely palliative.

- The next stage is often referral for one of several more invasive treatment options. This includes manipulation under anaesthesia (MUA) followed by several months of intensive physical therapy, or, if the problem is severe, more invasive surgery. The risks associated with MUA include fracture of the humerus, tendon rupture and nerve (brachial plexus) injury. As recently as November 2000 clinical trials showed that none of the above treatments give consistently reproducible success.

- Other surgical procedures include distension arthrography, where fluid is forced into the shrunken synovial bag; this is followed by several weeks of intensive physical therapy. Also diagnostic arthroscopy may be utilised and while 'inside' the shoulder the surgeon may try to treat the condition. If all of these fail, in severe cases total shoulder replacement (similar to hip replacement) may be performed.

what is happening inside my shoulder joint?

The causes of frozen shoulder syndrome are still poorly understood. About 50% seem to stem from an injury to the shoulder (such as a fall on an outstretched arm) and these are called secondary frozen shoulders. But 50% of the time they appear for no apparent reason, and these are called primary frozen shoulders. Although we don't know why they happen we do know a lot about what goes on inside the frozen shoulder.

As we have seen, the shoulder is a modified ball and socket joint. The ball is at the top of the arm bone (humerus) and the socket is a shallow cup on the end of the scapula (shoulder blade). This is a good design to give mobility to the shoulder joint but it makes it inherently unstable. To improve the stability of the shoulder, a cuff of four muscles (called the rotator cuff) braces the joint, as well as a complex plethora of tough internal ligaments.

Surrounding the gleno-humeral joint (shoulder joint) is a bag called the capsule. When the arm is raised above the head, this capsule is fully stretched, and when the arm is lowered to the side, the capsule hangs down in a small pouch-like sack (plica). The synovial capsule contains up to 60ml of synovial fluid. This fluid helps to lubricate the joint and gives the joint surfaces nutrients for repair. Cells lining the joint membrane produce the synovial fluid. Internal cameras have shown that during the frozen phase the capsule may shrink to less than half its normal size.

In frozen shoulder syndrome (adhesive capsulitis), this small sack starts to stick to itself, hence the name of the condition. As it becomes sticky, the synovial fluid drains away and can often reduce to about 5ml. This makes the joint dry and crackly. The stickiness is brought on through massive localised inflammation. This inflammation spreads into other shoulder soft-tissues and can cause swelling in other shoulder sacks (bursae). It has been my experience that this situation may occur the other way around as well. Often a frozen shoulder results from a non-treated biceps tendonitis, or triceps tendonitis. Both the biceps and triceps tendon run into the ball and socket joint. The tendons, like the muscles, are covered by a cling film-like sheath, which gets inflamed and becomes swollen, so the tendon can no longer slide smoothly as the arm is moved. This quickly leads to a vicious circle. The tendons become even more swollen and night pain commences. There is very little free space inside the shoulder joint and all of the tendon sheaths eventually blend together; they are continuous. This means that thousands of microscopic cells of inflammation can easily make their way from sheath to sheath and eventually the whole shoulder becomes engulfed in a rapid and massive inflammatory cycle.

The nature of inflammation (or swelling) is that it feels worse for rest; this is why the pain is worse at night. Once the arm is moved around, the swelling becomes dissipated and the pain is reduced. That is why you feel better when you have moved the arm around at night. There are in fact two types of inflammation: acute and chronic. Acute inflammation is the type that happens if you twist your ankle; it rapidly swells then rapidly diminishes over about 72 hours. If we were to take a sample of the fluid from the ankle and send it to the laboratory, it would have a specific profile of cells. When we see this specific profile we call it acute inflammation. In the case of frozen shoulder, there is some acute inflammation, but unfortunately a more sinister type of inflammation is also at work. This is called chronic inflammation and it has a different cellular profile. The difference is that chronic inflammation lasts a lot longer than 72 hours; once it has started it seems to fester insidiously for months on end. As soon as it seems to be getting better, a small setback can trigger the whole process off again in a vicious circle. Anti-inflammatory drugs are extremely effective at reducing acute inflammation but less good with chronic. This is the same for steroid injections, which block the production of a key ingredient of inflammation called 'substance P' (prostaglandin). This partly explains why tablets and injections have only a limited effect on frozen shoulder syndrome.

In less than a week, inflammation spreads throughout the joint and the arm movements rapidly start to diminish. Within a few weeks, the arm becomes frozen and for many cannot be raised more than 50° in any direction (normal sideways and front–back movement is 180°). The muscles of the rotator cuff become weak and slowly start to waste away, leaving the arm to hang stiff and useless for months on end.

It is worth going back to the neurology at this point. Muscle wasting occurs so fast that it cannot possibly be due to lack of use. Other factors are in operation here, and they are more than likely neurological. This is also the case when someone breaks a bone. When the arm is broken, for example, the muscles waste away within hours; again, this is not a result of under-use, it is a neurological phenomenon. I believe this is all part of the sensory-motor feedback loop, which we discussed

earlier. The sensory feedback from the joint is attenuated and as a result the muscles rapidly start to waste away. This is probably the result of an inbuilt protective mechanism. In the case of a fracture, muscle wasting may occur rapidly so we are forced to avoid putting any weight through the joint. In the case of a frozen shoulder, however, what is a protective mechanism becomes a hindrance, and the arm muscles are held rigid, wasted and useless.

This then is what is happening inside your shoulder joint. It may sound depressing but as we have said the vast majority of cases do get better eventually, and once you have had it, it almost never comes back again (unless you are one of the 12% who unfortunate enough to get it on the other side).

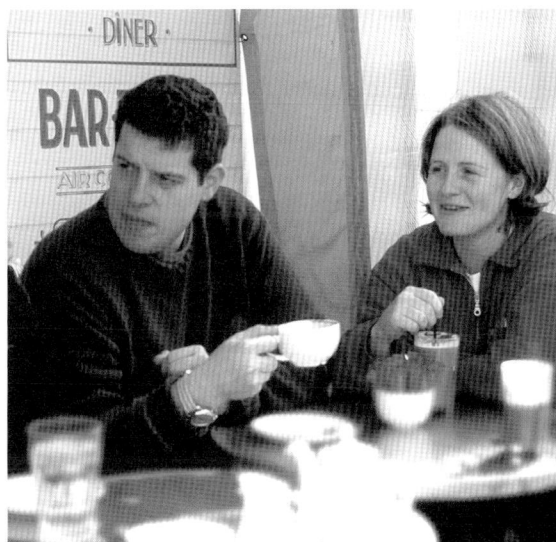

diabetes and the frozen shoulder

As we said earlier, frozen shoulder is much more common in diabetics; about 10-20% are affected (compared to 2-5% of the general population). It is not clear why this should be the case but experimental studies have shown that the soft tissues of the shoulder are stiffer than normal. All muscle fibres are 'packed' within other tissue called parenchyma. This packing substance is made of collagen. Collagen helps to make up the elastic component of the skin and muscles (as we get older our skin wrinkles as a result of decreased collagen production). US doctors NA Friedman and MM LaBan published a paper in 1989 in which they put forward two theories as to why frozen shoulder is more common in those suffering with diabetes.

Theory 1

Because type I diabetics are unable to regulate their blood sugar levels naturally, there are many times during the day that the sugar levels may be high, which can lead to an accumulation of sugar-alcohol in the tissues. This sugar-alcohol is called sorbitol and it accumulates in the 'ground substance' of the connective tissues (collagen) where, because it has a higher osmotic pressure, it attracts water, making the tissues stiffer.

Theory 2

An alternative explanation has been put forward, whereby the properties of the collagen itself are attenuated. It has been suggested that the collagen becomes embedded with excess sugar called glycogen. This 'glycosylation' of collagen leads to more bonds and bridges being formed at a molecular level between collagen molecules, thus changing the internal structure of the collagen. This means that enzymes cannot efficiently replace normal collagen wear and tear, and the tissues get stiffer.

collagen

It may be interesting to note the way normal collagen is produced in our muscle tissues. Collagen is fibrous and is formed by cells called fibroblasts. These are boat-shaped cells that roam throughout all muscle tissues. They produce long chains of fibres that get randomly meshed and woven together within the fluid or 'ground-substance' that supports the muscle cells. The reason I am going into such detail is that these fibroblasts lead short but interesting lives. They wander through the tissue producing fibres at random, and move by putting out finger-like projections into the tissue. If this projection should meet the finger-like projection of another fibroblast on its travels, they join hands (or fingers) and start combing the random collagen into nice straight packets. They can then live for a few days. If they don't meet another fibroblast, they die within a few hours. Apart from being a sweet story, this factor may be implicated in frozen shoulder syndrome. It has been suggested that in an attempt to repair itself, the body produces more fibroblasts. This creates an unusual situation, because the arm is held stiff and still whilst at the same time more fibroblasts are brushing the collagen into rope like structures, further stiffening the tissue around the muscle fibres.

Your diagnosis

As already stated, it is best to see your own medical practitioner for a diagnosis of frozen shoulder syndrome as several other conditions may mimic it. I will, however, discuss how a frozen shoulder is differentially diagnosed, and how I diagnose it still further. This is necessary, because I have developed three slight variations in the treatment programme.

The diagnosis must be based on a thorough case history and on a thorough physical examination. I will run through the history that I ask of my own patients. You can fill it in yourself and then we will go through it together a bit later on. Keep this for your records; it will help to record on-going information.

Your case

You should have received a blank case history form with this book. We are now going to fill this form in together. In the next chapter I have presented a case history form with questions. I want you to write the answers to these questions on the blank history form.

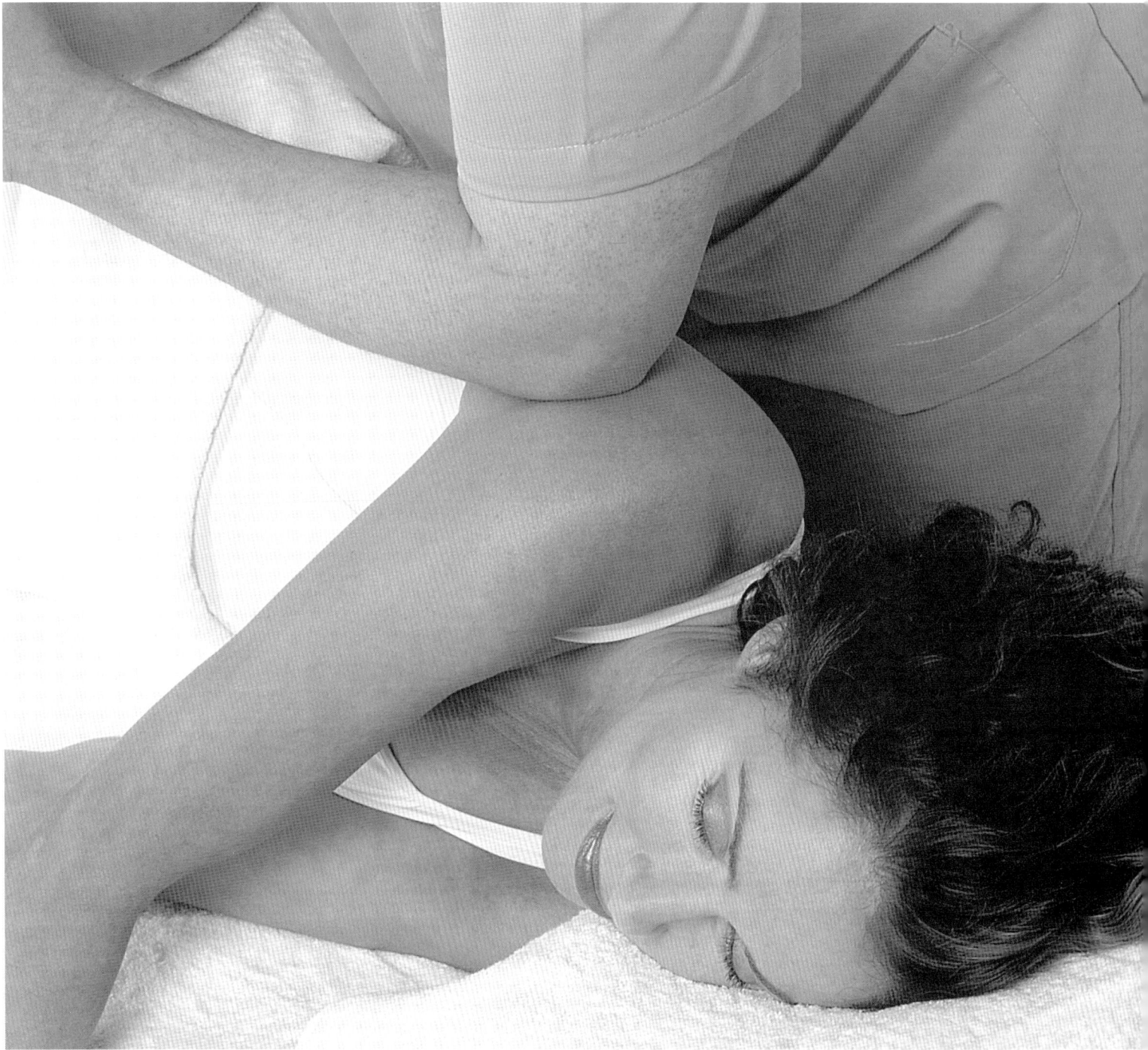

frozen shoulder case history

date _____   d.o.b (age) _____

name _____   G.P. _____

address _____   occupation _____

tel _____   hobbies/interests _____

email _____

complaint

which side?

where do you feel the pain?

is there night pain?

how many times do you wake at night?

do you get a sharp catching pain on certain movements?

which movements? (write them below under aggravating)

have you found anything that helps? (write under relieving)

is there a daily pattern to your pain?

history

how long have you had the symptoms?

how did it start? (traumatic or insidious)

have you had any medical investigations? who, what, where?

have you had any treatments?

how many and what type?

have they helped you?

aggravating   relieving   non-affecting

past medical history

accidents _____

illnesses _____

operations _____

family history

Diabetes? _____

Frozen shoulder? _____

Other? _____

general

how are your nails?

are they pitted or spooned? this might indicate anaemia

are your fingers like drum-sticks? this might indicate chest disease

are you right or left-handed?

systems

head and neck

general

trauma? headache? dizziness? fainting?

eyes

dry? prone to conjunctivitis?

ears

pain? discharge? tinitus, hearing change?

nose

sinus pain? discharge? nosebleeds? change in ability to smell?

throat

soreness? pain on swallowing? changes in speech?

neck

soreness? swellings?

respiratory

last chest film/x-ray? when and what did it show?

general

pain on breathing?

cough? sputum?

wheezing?

are you prone to chest infections?

exposure to irritants

occupational? habits? (smoking/alcohol)

circulatory

chest pain? breathlessness on exertion? _____

Raynaud's disease? _____

leg cramps or ankle swelling? _____

blood pressure? _____

are you passing water more frequently? _____

have you noticed you are more thirsty? _____

do you have pain or burning when you pass water? _____

have you been passing blood? _____

have you been passing water more than once per night? _____

any recent or sudden change in habit? _____

cystitis? _____

reproductive

male

have you had a venereal disease or non-specific urethritis? _____

have you noticed any testicle swellings? _____

do you have any prostate symptoms?

female

when was your last period? has the cycle length changed? _____

do you suffer with painful or heavy periods? _____

any irregularities e.g. discharge? _____

any breast swelling, nodules or tenderness? _____

musculosketal

any muscular weakness or pain? (other than in the shoulder) _____

any tremors? _____

neurological

headaches? fainting? seizures? _____

weakness? paralysis? _____

pins and needles? _____

haematopoietic

anaemia? _____

transfusions? _____

easy bruising or bleeding? _____

metabolic

excessive urination or thirst? _____

any growth or developmental changes? _____

any recent or rapid weight changes? _____

diet

any food allergies? _____

medication

any psychiatric medication? _____

other medication?

observations

side? right, left or both? _____

date												
flexion												
extension												
abduction												
external rotation												

soft tissues

can you detect any areas of tenderness or pain?
write them here or draw them if you like!

_____

_____

diagnosis (Please circle)

anterior

posterior

lateral

treatment plan

anterior only

posterior only

anterior and posterior

lateral only

antero-lateral

postero-Lateral

all three

any other comments

_____

_____

_____

_____

_____

_____

_____

_____

_____

_____

_____

_____

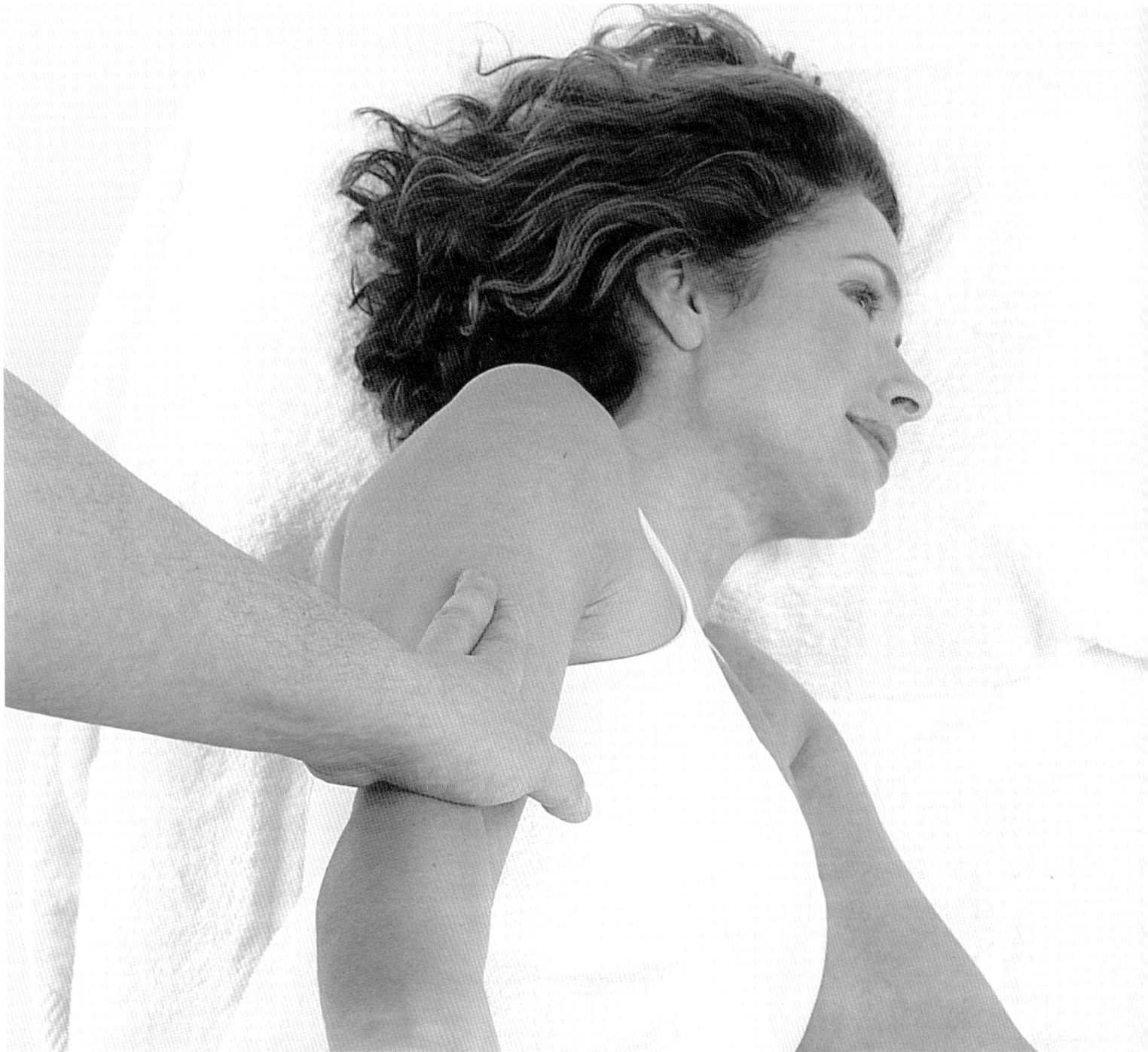

objectives

After studying this chapter, you should be able to:

- Use a goniometer
- Fill in your case history form
- Understand the differences between a typical anterior, posterior and lateral frozen shoulder
- Familiarise yourself with the pathological sieve
- Understand the process of differential diagnosis
- Familiarise yourself with examples of different types of frozen shoulder
- Analyse your case history
- Diagnose your type of frozen shoulder

This chapter provides examples of typical cases of frozen shoulder syndrome. They are used to illustrate the type of experiences that might be familiar to you. Remember that there are other types of problems that can mimic a frozen shoulder. If you are in any doubt as to your diagnosis, please consult your doctor.

Please note how the degrees of movement have been filled in. These are typical for the various types of frozen shoulder syndrome.

goniometry

You should have received a goniometer with this book. This instrument allows you to measure shoulder movement accurately. It is easy to use: place it by the joint where you are measuring movement; keep one part toward the floor and read off the angle between the floor and the affected arm. I measure passive movements which means I lift the arm up to its maximum range.

Abduction, flexion and extension all involve the gleno-humeral joint, so the movement should be measured at that joint.

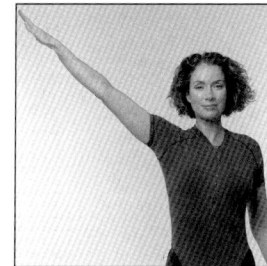

135° Abduction

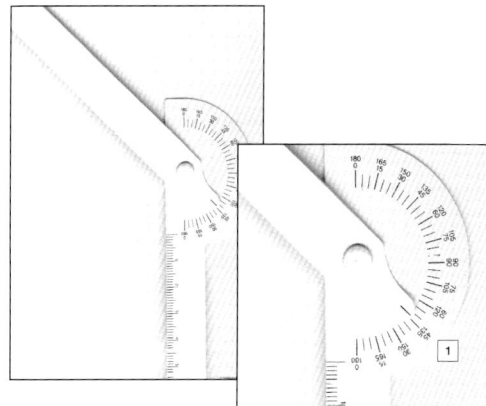

1. Read off the degrees of movement (angle) between the floor and the affected arm

example 1 freezing

Female UK Age 54 Artist

complains of: Left shoulder pain, severe aching and discomfort 'inside' the joint. Pain radiating down the outside of the upper arm. Severe night pain especially if lying on the left side. Can awake several times during the night – occasionally with some numbness in the hand. Pain is getting worse. Stiffness of the arm and shoulder. Aggravated by reaching behind, doing hair, putting on a bra. Severe sharp pain on reaching for certain objects – can last 2–3 minutes.

history: 4-month history. Started for no apparent reason. However, patient had recently started playing golf. Saw a chiropractor four times who took x-rays of the spine (not effective). Saw a cranial osteopath five times (some short-term relief). Went to GP who sent her to an orthopaedic consultant – x-rays. Nothing abnormal diagnosed (NAD). Diagnosed as a severe frozen shoulder and advised either arthroscopy (micro-surgery) or to wait for two and a half years.

past medical history: None

family history: None

general impressions: Otherwise fit and well; right-handed

systems: Slight bowel complaint, Raynaud's syndrome, panic attacks and asthma

medicines: HRT and Ventolin™

date	16/2	22/2	1/3	8/3	14/3	22/3	13/4	18/4
flexion (°) *	120	130	140	145	145	155	165	175
extension (°)	35	40	50	55	55	60	70	70
abduction (°)	80	100	115	135	140	145	160	175
external rotation (°)	45	45	50	55	60	60	70	70
change in pain (%)		5	70	70	75	99	99	99

*These numbers show the angle measured in degrees using the goniometer

diagnosis: Phase 1-2 **anterior** frozen shoulder

example 2 frozen

Female UK Age 61 Psychotherapist

complains of: Left shoulder pain. Stiffness of the arm and shoulder. Some night pain (but less than it used to be) mainly if sleeps on the left side. Pain at end of range of movement. Weakness and pain in neck and shoulders. Aggravated by reaching behind the back and putting on a bra.

history: 11-month history. Awoke with left arm above head in pain (often sleeps in this position). Very severe pain and restriction for first four months. Saw a chiropractor four times who took x-rays of the spine (not effective). Saw GP who diagnosed a frozen shoulder and gave one steroid injection (not effective). Two months later he sent her to an orthopaedic consultant who gave another steroid injection and advised physical therapy, 10 sessions (mild relief).

past medical history: Hip replacement, disc problem in the low back

family history: None

general impressions: Otherwise fit and well; right-handed

systems: Heart arrhythmia, occasional palpitations, acid indigestion, bloating, stress incontinence

medicines: HRT, propanalol, Zantac™, NSAIDs

date	15/3	30/3	11/4	10/5	23/5	6/6	20/6
flexion (°)	115	125	140	155	160	170	180
extension (°)	35	40	50	55	60	65	70
abduction (°)	85	95	125	145	155	165	180
external rotation (°)	30	35	45	55	60	65	70
change in pain (%)		5	80	95	95	99	99

diagnosis: Phase 2 **anterior** frozen shoulder

example 3 thawing

Male The Netherlands Age 44 Surveyor

complains of: Left shoulder pain; constant background ache. Stiffness of the arm and shoulder. Some night pain if sleeps on the right side. Pain at end of range of movement can be severe. Aggravated by 'reaching for hip pocket'. Sharp pain on certain movements; pain at the top-back of the arm.

history: 18-month history. No apparent reason. Saw GP after three months who diagnosed a frozen shoulder gave a three steroid injections (limited relief). Six months later sent to an orthopaedic surgeon who diagnosed a 'frozen shoulder', 'rotator cuff damage' and 'sub-acromial impingement syndrome'. He gave another steroid injection and did an MRI scan which confirmed the diagnosis. Had five months of physical therapy (44 sessions, mild relief). Had an arthroscopic operation and a manipulation under anaesthesia. Symptoms worsened, had a second MRI scan. Advised that he would need 'nerve block' injections to ease the pain.

past medical history: Achilles tendon repair, disc problems in low back

family history: Frozen shoulder

general impressions: Otherwise fit and well; right-handed

systems: Nothing abnormal recorded

medicines: NSAIDs

date	12/10	26/10	9/11	21/11	7/12	16/12	20/6
flexion (°)	95	125	145	155	165	180	180
extension (°)	50	50	50	50	55	65	70
abduction (°)	85	115	125	150	160	180	180
external rotation (°)	50	50	55	55	65	70	70
change in pain (%)		5	5	30	40	99	99

diagnosis: Phase 3 **anterior** + **posterior** frozen shoulder

example 4

Female UK Age 58 Secretary

complains of: Right shoulder pain. Severe night pain when lying down at night. Weakness and pain in neck and shoulders. Pain comes in waves and can be severe. When pain is bad patient feels sick. If severe pain, can extend to arm and hand.

history: 6-month history. Symptoms gradually getting worse. Not seen GP. Advised to go to my clinic by a friend. No real daily pattern.

past medical history: Hip replacement, disc problem in low back

family history: Bowel cancer

general impressions: Otherwise fit and well; right-handed

systems: Abdominal bloating and wind, fatty stools (steatorrhoea), decreased appetite for fatty foods. Duodenal ulcer.

medicines: HRT, Zantac™, painkillers.

examination: Revealed shoulder pain on pressing the upper right abdomen (Murphy's sign).

date						
flexion (°)						
extension (°)						
abduction (°)						
external rotation (°)						
change in pain (%)						

diagnosis: Cholecystitis (gall stones)

differential diagnosis of frozen shoulder syndrome – what else could it be?

As stated earlier, many different conditions can mimic a frozen shoulder. It is important to know this. Don't be alarmed, as most of the conditions below are rarely a cause of frozen shoulder. However, if you are in any doubt at all, please consult your doctor; it's better to be safe.

When I look at any physical problem that presents in my clinic, I always sift the information gleaned from the case history and examination through what is called a pathological sieve. This acts as a filter and allows us to think laterally at the same time. I'm afraid I will have to use some medical terms; some of these terms are explained in the index, others can be got from any good medical dictionary such as Tabers medical dictionary (or from the Internet).

congenital

Errors in joint formation, lack or deformation of cartilaginous labrum, congenital disorders of cervical spine

degenerative

Osteoporosis, osteopaenia, degenerative arthritis, disc degeneration of the cervical spine, cervical myelopathy, cervical bar formation, osteophytic impingement of cervical nerve root, bony spur growth, Parkinson's disease

metabolic

Pagets disease, osteomalacia, gouty arthritis, hyperparathyroidism, polymyalgia rheumatica (GCA) haemophiliac bleed, hypercalcinosis, pseudo-gout

functional

Sub-acromial bursitis, biceps tendonitis, rotator cuff tear, biceps rupture, arthritis of the acromi-clavicular joint, shoulder-hand syndrome, thoracic outlet syndrome, heart attack, gastric ulcer, cholycystitis or cholelithiasis (gall bladder for right shoulder), stroke

infective

Osteomalacia, joint infection, septic arthritis

neoplastic

Myeloma, osteosarcoma (rare), primary bone tumour, secondary bone tumour (metastasis from prostate, lung, breast, thyroid, bone, skin etc) pancoast tumour, stomach cancer (for left shoulder)

reticulo-endothelial

Osteochondromatosis, monostotic arthritis secondary to Reiter's syndrome, Beçets syndrome

traumatic

Clavicle fracture, spiral fracture of the humerus, fracture of humeral head, displaced fracture, untreated shoulder dislocation, avascular-necrosis, cervical spine disc, prolapse with nerve root compression

analysing your case history

I will start by giving you the kind of history I would expect to hear in my own practice, because frozen shoulder has such a well-documented natural history I would expect your case to fit into one of the patterns I will describe. As we go along, I will make some suggestions as to how I might diagnose your frozen shoulder. If your case is radically different, it may be worth consulting your own doctor for further investigation.

We will now explore how to fill in the supplied blank case history form with your case history.

filling in the case history, page 1

age: The age is likely to be between 40 and 70 (although I have seen exceptions).

sex: It is more common in females aged 40-60

occupation: There doesn't seem to be a correlation with occupation.

hobbies: Golf, tennis and swimming are often reported as the trigger of symptoms.

complaint: As stated previously, the non-dominant arm is more likely to be affected. Patients often complain of pain and stiffness running down the side of the upper arm in a band. This is slightly odd because there are no muscles here, only fascial tissue. (In fact it is actually the fascial tissue that causes pain. As you will see later, it becomes tethered, fibrous and lumpy.)

You may get a severe sharp pain on moving your arm without thinking; this can last for a few minutes. This is probably from a grossly inflamed biceps tendon. This would indicate to me that you might have an **anterior** frozen shoulder.

You may have pain and stiffness at the back of the arm and shoulder. This would indicate to me a **posterior** frozen shoulder.

You may have pain radiating into the forearm, hand and/or wrist (reflex sympathetic dystrophy).

You may have a constant 'deep burning ache' within the shoulder.

Your main pain may be located just below the acromion-clavicular joint at the upper outside part of the arm. This would indicate to me a **lateral** frozen shoulder.

You may very well have a combination of all the above. You will probably have night pain, especially if you lie on the affected side. In my experience, most people have night pain. It can be especially severe in the freezing phase, but can be severe in the frozen and thawing phases. Generally speaking, the night pain does tend to lessen with time. Patients in the frozen and thawing phases tend to have night pain after a few hours of lying down. (In fact I have found that the degree of night pain is a good indicator of treatment progress.) I have only ever seen a few cases where there is no night pain within the first ten months. I have known patients who have been unable to sleep properly for months on end. This obviously leads to exhaustion and fatigue which can cause its own set of problems. Hopefully, sleep should be one of the first things to improve if you follow my treatment plan.

You will almost certainly also have stiffness of the shoulder. This varies in degree but movement can sometimes be very restricted. Sometimes patients have no more than a few degrees of movement in any direction. Often, when people lift their arms up sideways, they find that they have to cheat by bending the whole spine.

actions that aggravate frozen shoulder

Putting on or taking off a jumper or coat, reaching for the back pocket, combing the hair, reaching towards the back seat of the car, changing gears, reaching to unlock the back door of the car, picking up a case, reaching behind the back to do up the bra, cleaning up after going to the toilet.

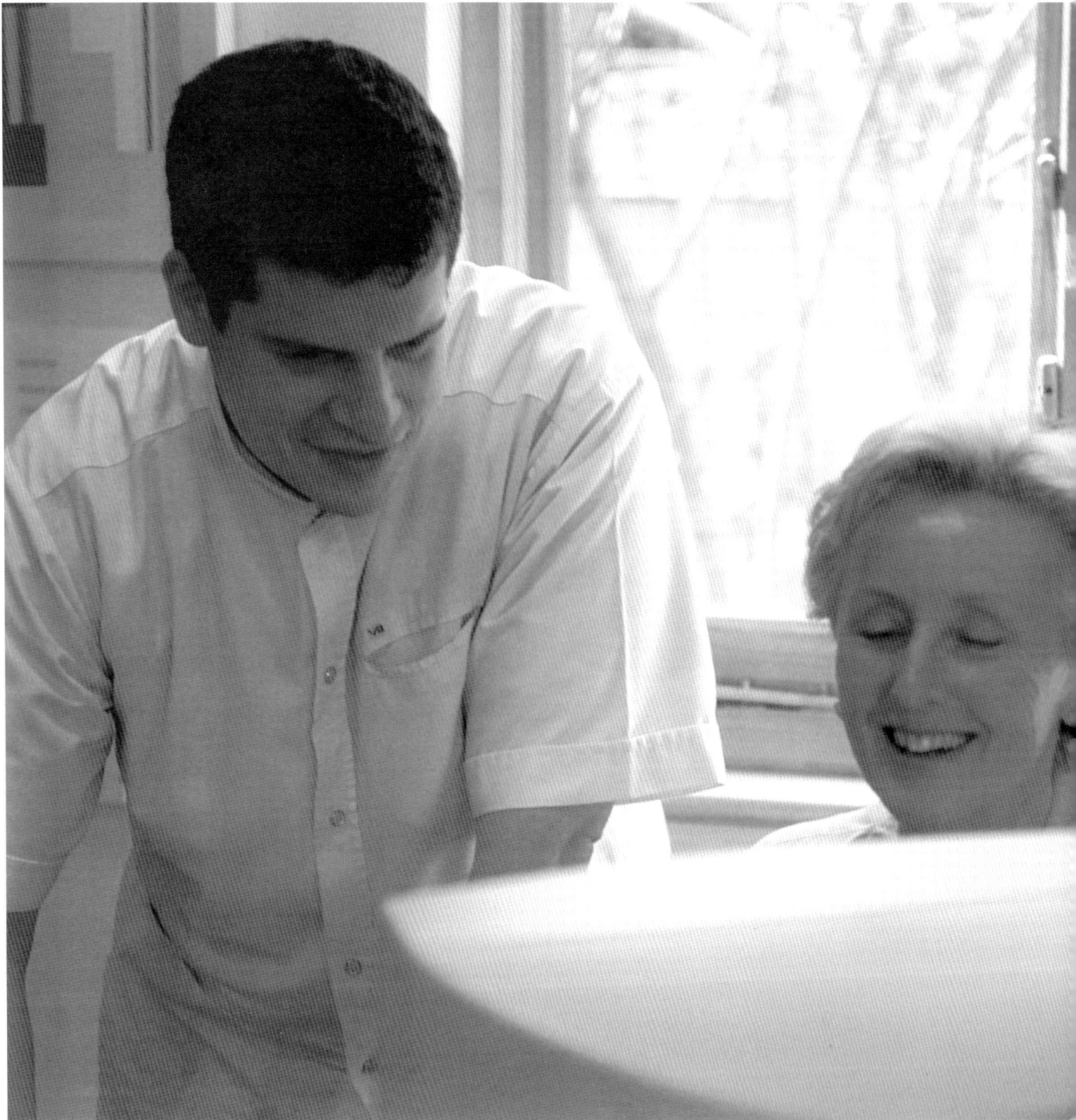

pain relief

Usually there is very little that helps a frozen shoulder. Occasionally medication such as NSAIDs may relieve the pain, as will a hot bath, but it has been my experience that relief is temporary. Often patients say that there is absolutely nothing that helps.

The daily pattern, if there is one, tends to be of pain at night, which eases slightly during the day, or, in the frozen and thawing phases no real pain unless pushed to the limits of movement.

history

As stated previously, frozen shoulder has three phases. As a rule of thumb you can think of the freezing phase lasting for the first six months, the frozen phase from seven to 4 months and the thawing phase from 15 months onwards. Which phase are you in?

Often severe cases of frozen shoulder follow a trauma to the shoulder. I have often heard people say that their frozen shoulder started from an ache after swimming, doing a sport (such as golf) or gardening, the kind of ache you think will just go away but doesn't, and after a few weeks the whole shoulder seems to stiffen.

In women I have often found that symptoms come on for no reason at all. This can be the case for men as well. In my opinion, there is probably a build up of small repetitive tears in the muscles, leading to micro-bleeds. These tears tend to repair themselves at night when the shoulder is not being used.

Frozen shoulder sometimes occurs after an emotional trauma such as divorce or the loss of a loved one.

In a typical **anterior** frozen shoulder, the pain tends to begin with a biceps tendonitis. This usually presents as an ache at the front of the shoulder and a sharp catching sensation with certain movements. I have found that even with treatment, biceps tendonitis can lead to a frozen shoulder. Untreated biceps tendonitis will almost certainly progress this way. My method for treating the **anterior** frozen shoulder seems to work extremely well for the treatment of biceps tendonitis as well. (This is the most common presentation in my own practice, accounting for about 70% of cases; it is also the easiest to treat.)

In a typical **posterior** frozen shoulder, the main symptomatic area is at the top of the triceps muscle. Often in this case I will diagnose a 'triceps tendonitis'. To the best of my knowledge, I was the first to discover this condition. The pain and stiffness seem to come on more rapidly in a **posterior** frozen shoulder. The pain is less 'catchy' and patients tend to report stiffness as their main symptom. (This is a less common presentation – about 20% of cases. It responds well to treatment but tends to require a deeper and more vigorous approach.)

A **lateral** frozen shoulder tends to start with a fall on the shoulder. It can also be a sequel to an 'impingement syndrome', such as sub-acromial bursitis or a bony spur (formation) within the joint. The pain tends to be more at the tip of the shoulder and movement seems to become very restricted.
It generally starts with a catching pain in the shoulder as the arm is taken above the head and backwards in a circle. These tend to be the most severe cases. I have also seen **lateral** frozen shoulders as a result of failed shoulder surgery. I rarely see them presenting on their own because they usually occur with an **anterior** or **posterior** frozen shoulder. (They account for about 10% of the cases I see; they tend to be the most severe and respond more slowly to treatment. This is because the inflammation lies in a position that is difficult to reach.)

medical investigations

These include x-rays, MRI scans, CT scans and radioisotope scans, arthrography (injecting dye into the shoulder joint) or arthroscopy (surgery). X-rays are useful for ruling out other suspected conditions such as arthritis, they often show nothing at all. If they do show anything, it is usually a decreased joint space, calcium deposits and/or minimal arthritic changes in the bones (in long-standing cases). Sometimes your doctor may do a blood test to rule out any other conditions. More often than not these investigations show up nothing abnormal.

who, what, where?

Most patients start by going to their GP, who might then prescribe anti-inflammatory drugs. If these do not work (which is usually the case) the GP may give a steroid injection or refer you to a specialist (orthopaedic surgeon or rheumatologist). Steroid injections have been shown to help the situation somewhat but they rarely 'cure' a frozen shoulder. It is not advisable to have more than three injections. The specialist may then send you to hospital for further investigations. S/he may then offer further steroid injections or send you to a physical therapist or perhaps advise surgery.

The most common operation is manipulation under anaesthesia (MUA), which is usually offered in cases of long-standing frozen shoulder. This procedure, proposed originally by Duplay, is dramatic and has its critics. You will be given a general anaesthetic and the arm is then bent and small jerky movements are made in various directions to 'tear apart' the adhesions. The patient is then sent off for immediate post-operative physiotherapy. The risks attached to it should be mentioned. These are: fracture of the humerus, dislocation of the shoulder, injury to major nerve groups (brachial plexus) and, of course, reactions to the general anaesthetic. There are conflicting results from MUA studies, ranging from 90% showing some improvement to 80% showing little or no improvement; a lot depends on who performs the operation. It is not uncommon to have over 20 sessions of physical therapy after an MUA.

Some patients go directly to a physical therapist. These are osteopaths, physiotherapists, massage therapists, acupuncturists, chiropractors etc. It is not uncommon to have more than 12 sessions. The most I have seen was a woman from Saudi Arabia who had endured 144 physical therapy sessions and was still no better. In my opinion, the way physical therapists treat frozen shoulders often makes the patient worse, especially if they try to force the arm to its limits. Any of those who have had this type of treatment will know what I mean. Generally physical therapy does not seem to help much during the first ten months; it may be of use after this. I would like to point out here that analysis of every case I have treated with the Niel-Asher Technique™ showed that 82% of cases recovered fully and a further 8% improved by 70% or more with an average of seven treatment sessions.

past medical history

Some details of your past medical history may be relevant to your frozen shoulder. This list is not exhaustive. If you have had any of the accidents, illnesses or operations mentioned below or you are worried about any others, please contact your own doctor before using the Niel-Asher Technique™.

The factors that may be relevant are listed opposite.

accidents

- Trauma to arm or shoulder including fracture or dislocation
- Trauma or dislocation of the collar-bone (clavicle)
- Falls on an outstretched arm
- Previous shoulder surgery
- Problems with the neck
- Road accident

illnesses

- Polymyalgia rheumatica (PMR)
- Diabetes mellitus
- Lung, breast, skin or prostate cancer
- Pancoast tumour
- Paget's disease
- Myocardial Infarction
- Parkinson's disease

operations

- Previous shoulder surgery
- Neck surgery
- Immobilisation (splinting) following wrist, hand or arm surgery

family history

There is no conclusive evidence that frozen shoulder is an inherited condition. However, there may be a history of diabetes in the family and occasionally a frozen shoulder is the first sign of diabetes.

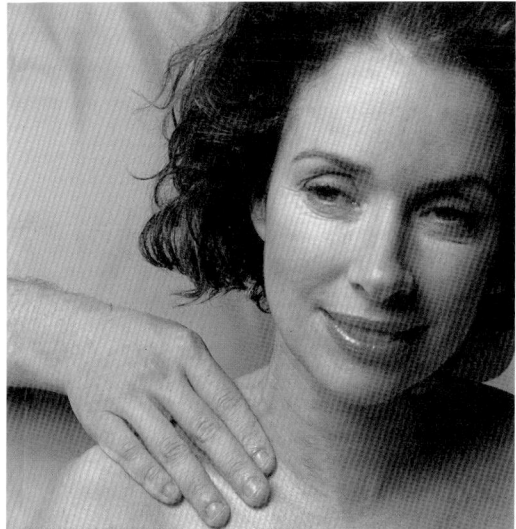

filling in the case history, pages 2 and 3

systems

If you answer yes to any of the questions below and are worried, please contact your doctor. Apart from the medical conditions mentioned above, there is no exact correlation between a frozen shoulder and any other medical complaint. The main things to look out for, however, are the following:

respiratory

Are you a smoker? Do you have a constant wheeze? Has one of your eyelids started to droop? Have the muscles around your thumb wasted away? Have you been coughing up blood? Have you been losing weight for no reason? A yes to any of these will need further investigation.

circulatory

There may be a relationship between frozen shoulder and Raynaud's syndrome. Do you suffer from cold hands and feet? Do you suffer from chest pain? A yes to either of these may need further investigation.

gastrointestinal

Do you find that you are avoiding fatty foods? Have your stools changed colour or consistency? Do you cough up blood? A yes to any of these may need further investigation.

genitourinary

Are you passing water more frequently? Are you having to pass water more than once per night? Has the colour or consistency of your urine changed? Are you excessively thirsty? Do you suffer with prostate problems? A yes to any of these may need further investigation.

reproductive - male

Have you ever suffered with non-specific urethritis? Have you noticed any swellings in your testes? A yes may need further investigation.

Don't forget, a yes to any of the other system questions may require further medical investigation.

filling in the case history, page 4 and 5

Along with this book you should have received a goniometer. This is a type of ruler that allows you to measure the degrees of movement of the shoulder joint. If you look at the case history examples above, you will see that I have filled them in. Here is another example of a table that I have filled in.

date	12/10	26/10	9/11	21/11	7/12	16/12
flexion (°)	95	125	145	155	165	180
extension (°)	50	50	50	50	55	65
abduction (°)	85	115	125	150	160	180
external rotation (°)	50	50	55	55	65	70

As you can see I have filled in the date of each treatment and degrees of movement for flexion, extension, abduction and external rotation. I would urge you to do this yourself as it gives a good indication of treatment progress. In my own practice, having measured shoulder movement, I either take a photograph or a video clip of shoulder movement at the beginning of each treatment session; you may want to do the same. To use the goniometer, move the arms of the goniometer apart to match the angle at which the arm can be raised and then read off the result. Record the results in the boxes. Do not push the arm above its maximum stretch, as this will traumatise it. However, sometimes in long-standing cases you may find that there is more movement if the arm is helped up than is possible on your own. This may be due to the wasting and weakness of the shoulder muscles which have not been used properly for some time.

flexion: Maximum 180°

extension: Maximum 70–80°   (see chapter 1)

abduction: Maximum 180°

external rotation: Maximum 75°

your diagnosis

Using the history and examination we can now arrive at your diagnosis. If you are unsure which type of frozen shoulder you have, do not worry as the three treatment programmes have a lot of overlap. The treatment method I am presenting in this book is for the **anterior** presentation. Following this protocol in all cases this should improve your pain and range of motion. If you suspect you have a **posterior** and/or **lateral** diagnosis, following the 5 step programme is a great place to start; but I highly recommend you seek treatment from a qualified Niel-Asher technique practitioner (see www.frozenshoulder.com).

the Niel-Asher technique™

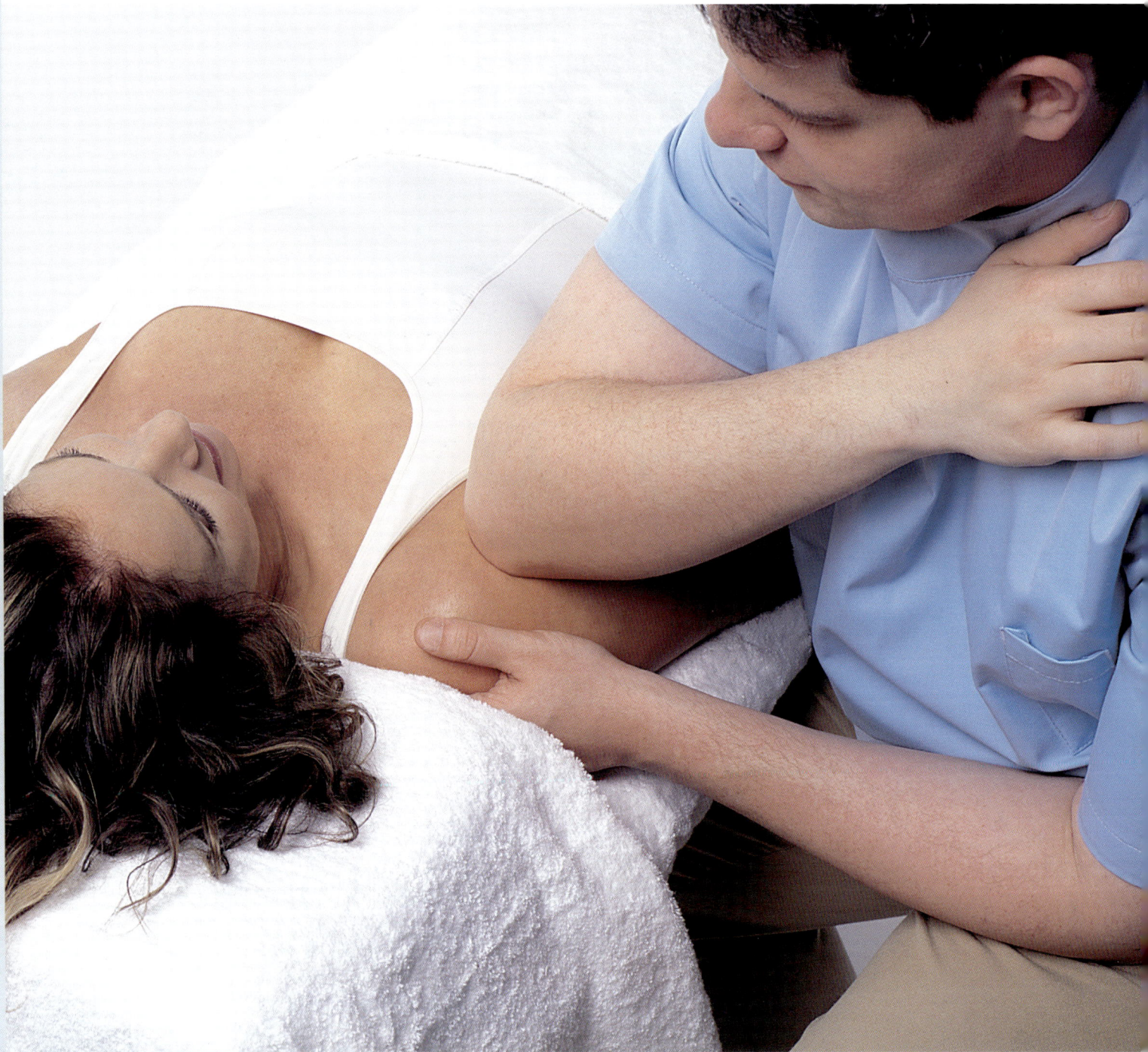

objectives

After studying this chapter, you should be able to:

- Understand the Niel-Asher Technique™
- Understand trigger point release
- Understand why frozen shoulder is more common in diabetics
  This chapter includes:
- Frequently asked questions (FAQs)
- Do the Niel-Asher Technique™ in steps

the Niel-Asher technique™

I have developed my unique approach to the treatment of frozen shoulder syndrome over the past six years. It all started when a family friend developed the condition in 1996. After many physiotherapy sessions and two operations she was no better; in fact she was worse. When she came to me I did not hold out a lot of hope, but she was desperate, even suicidal, with the pain. This got me thinking about the condition and researching methods for treatment. When I found none, I decided to invent my own. I have treated hundreds of patients with my method from all over the world, and have about a 90% success rate for frozen shoulder.

Having gone through your case history, you should now have an idea of whether you have got an **anterior**, **posterior** or **lateral** frozen shoulder. As previously stated, you may have a mixture of the above. I will describe the way I work and then present the technique for the anterior presentation with pictures and diagrams. Anterior cases represent 70% of all cases; the remaining 30% all have an anterior component.

The technique must be performed in a specific sequence. In fact, it is the order that is of utmost importance because the technique 'fools' the body into healing itself by working one group of muscles against another in a choreographed sequence. It works a bit like a recipe.

The Niel-Asher technique™ is a 'natural' method utilising the body's own healing mechanisms. It is not uncommon to experience soreness after treatment, which may last for 48 to 72 hours. This is a sign of the body healing itself and is not a sign of failure. If you are worried, you can stop the treatment and use some anti-inflammatory medication (see under advice, page 85). In my experience the first few treatments can be the most painful, because they work on already painful and inflamed tissues. As the range of movement returns and the tissues start to normalise, treatment becomes less painful, until eventually there should be no pain at all. Make sure you drink plenty of fresh water after treatment as this helps to 'flush' away some of the toxins released by/through treatment.

please note

If your symptoms are aggravated for more than 72 hours following treatment, please stop using this method for a couple of weeks and then try again; or perhaps seek advice from a qualified Niel-Asher technique practitioner.

trigger point release

what is a trigger point?

A trigger point is a nodule within a muscle where some of the muscle fibres have contracted into a ball. Pressing it in the right way has the effect of a short cut to relaxing the whole muscle. In this way you can release muscles in spasm without having to spend hours in massage, and irritating them further. The trigger point is located within the hot zone (see opposite).

direct and indirect

There are two components to my technique. One involves sustained direct pressure on (sometimes painful) tissues in a specific order. The other involves working on other tissue structures sometimes away from the painful areas. Although these tissues are directly linked to your shoulder pain, this is the indirect part of the technique. It is not uncommon and in fact is somewhat desirable that pressure on indirect tissues reproduces or mimics the underlying symptoms.

- After any deep tissue pressure, apply some gentle massage to the area. This gives a different type of stimulation to the brain, which reinforces the message from the deep tissue work.

- Then follow by gently moving the bent arm in ever increasing circles – but this should not cause pain.

frequently asked questions

what equipment do I need?

You need a bed (or a couch) though sometimes a table with some padding will suffice. Always lie on the good arm (or better arm first if both are affected).

what handhold do I use?

I use my elbow for treating the pressure points. This is because it allows me to generate more force. This is something that you can try, but at the beginning you may tend to slip off the painful bits. Instead try using your thumb reinforced with your other hand behind it.

how much pressure do I use?

This is something that comes with experience but as a rule of thumb the more painful the tissue the slower and deeper the pressure. In all cases, the key is to work slowly and thoroughly.

what if I bruise?

Bruising should not occur if you follow the instructions. I have found that it is not the depth of treatment that will cause a bruise but usually pressure applied too quickly. Try to feel the muscles and tender nodules beneath the skin. Arnica creams and tablets have been shown to reduce the incidence and severity of bruising. Unfortunately some people bruise more easily than others, especially if they are on certain medication. Some medication may exacerbate the tendency to bruise.

what is the direction of force?

This is an interesting question. I have tried wherever possible to indicate the direction of force on the pictures. The direction of force varies slightly from person to person. In general, the aim is to reproduce the painful symptoms. When you find the painful nodules, hold them with a sustained pressure, and change or vary the direction of force. I usually take the pressure clockwise until I hit the exact right point. Note the effects that this has on the pain.

hot zone

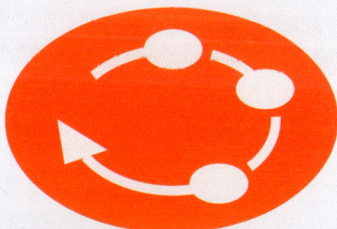

Direction of pressure within zone

It often amazes me that a slight change in the direction of the pressure can cause a totally different pain elsewhere. We want to find the direction of pressure that, where possible, reproduces the exact pain that you feel.

what is fascia?

This is an important structure that I believe is worth spending a few moments on. Fascia is also known as connective tissue and is clear but fibrous. It is modified (superficial or deep) according to where it is in the body but it is a bit like cling film. If you eat chicken, you may well be aware of the superficial fascia. It lies under the skin and is a tough transparent (cling-film like) tissue layer.

Most living organisms have fascia. It abounds in plant life. Here it is often not a tough clear layer (although it is the clear stuff that lies between onion layers) but is often dense and white and called pith. To explain fascia to my patients, I find it easier to think of oranges. In an orange the skin is a modified layer of fascia. Below the skin surrounding the segments is the white pith; this is also fascia. The segments of the orange are contained in clear bag-like structures and are fascial. Then if you look carefully the juice is held in tiny bags, these are also fascial. In humans, fascia is ubiquitous: it covers

and surrounds our organs; it covers the muscles; and it acts as the 'packing tissue' throughout the body. The capsules of the joints and the ligaments are also constructed from fascia. Even bone is (essentially) fascia that has become impregnated with calcium potassium and magnesium salts.

The fascia we are interested in covers the muscles like an envelope. It is like plastic when it is injured or damaged it becomes shorter, condensed and tighter. This is what gives it the nodular feel underneath the skin.

nodules are trigger points

In both chronic and acute shoulder pain, much of the fascia begins to tighten. As stated earlier, fascia condenses where it is damaged. It 'shrink wraps' various structures. The capsule tightens and is poorly repaired and the enveloping fascia that wraps around muscles tenses, especially where there is wasting. Lack of use fuels this fascial condensation and this is particularly pronounced in the diabetic frozen shoulder, or chronic frozen shoulder. There may be underlying fascial tightening in all shoulder structures, especially in long-standing cases. Wear and tear of all shoulder structures can be clearly seen from the age of 30 which is earlier than in almost any other joint (due mainly to the degree of flexibility and the amount we use our shoulders, arms and hands).

what creams or lotions should I use?

In general, it is better to avoid oils as they may cause you to slide off the pressure points once you have found them. I use plain Nivea™ cream. Alternatively, arnica cream or plain aqueous cream will do. Also petroleum gel or massage oil may be used, if you have a lanolin allergy.

is the treatment painful?

The treatment can be painful, but it should be no worse than what you are currently experiencing. The pain from this technique is a type of therapeutic pain. By reproducing your painful symptoms your partner/ therapist is sending positive affirmations to your brain, which allows it to think differently about your problem. Try not to be afraid of the pain, it should ease each time you are treated. It helps to breath deeply into the pain; try to melt it away with deep breathing. Do not pull away from it; remember pain is a signal, within a few minutes of sustained pressure the pain will rapidly ease.

can a partner really treat me?

There are clearly inherent difficulties in intimate friends/ partners (essentially) inflicting pain one on the other. This is why, of course, doctors are not encouraged to treat their own family. Now there is no way round this, realistically, if you want to get the maximum relief from this technique, but you must focus on the fact that this technique will help you. I am a firm believer that partners should touch and treat each other where possible, but clearly for some of you there may be some boundary and consent issues. If you are unhappy about working with a loved one talk it through and perhaps ask someone else to work on you. Also remember that this technique can be quite tiring for the person doing it so be patient with them and give them plenty of encouragement and feedback.

to get the best results!

The technique works through a cumulative effect that is, a little at a time. It may take two or three sessions to start seeing results but be patient. Remember you are re-programming the way the brain thinks about the shoulder. Have faith in the technique – it really does work. Do not charge in and force the technique every day. Give a few days break in between sessions (preferably four days). It is better to go slowly and respectfully than to force and rush this method.

anterior, leosterior or lateral?

In this guide I have presented my treatment for the **anterior** frozen shoulder. This is the most common presentation. If your problem is other than this I recommend that you see a qualified Niel-Asher technique™ therapist.

A list of qualified practitioners is available on my website www.frozenshoulder.com

the 1-2-3-4-5

My technique involves a combination of five simple components. This is what I call the 1-2-3-4-5. Other steps are added, but these form the basis of the technique. These five procedures MUST be done in the right order.

I would suggest that you begin with the generalised shoulder procedure. It introduces your hands to the patient. The touch should be firm and confident but not painful. It should feel good for you and for the patient. As a rule, if it feels good for you it feels good for the patient.

generalised shoulder procedure

This is best performed before and after each treatment session.

Start with the patient in a sitting position, perhaps on a stool. Feel the upper fibres of the trapezius muscle, taking note of the nodules beneath the skin. It is worth noting that, with a long-standing shoulder problem, the neck will have suffered somewhat. Often you will find an especially tough area half way between the neck and the shoulder. Massage the area gonorally and then put deep pressure through one of these painful spots. Build up the pressure slowly until you have hit the pain zone. If this is too much to bear, then reduce the pressure but do not pull away entirely from the painful point. The initial reaction is to pull away but stay with it until it is no longer painful. This can take anywhere up to two minutes. The pain will diminish, even on very tender areas. Ask the patient to focus on their breathing and visualise the tender point melting away.

It is important that you do not come away too soon as this will cause the tissues to tense against you. This type of sustained deep pressure has many effects, some of which have been discussed earlier. Other effects include:

- A type of numbing of the treated area
- Attenuation of the pain feedback pathways
- Stretching tight structures – which will have an indirect effect on all tissue structures
- Opening out the plastic fascial bag
- Stimulating the blood supply to clear away debris and toxins
- The release of powerful pain killing agents called endorphins

Be careful not to press too hard; you want to be in the 'painful' zone but no more than that. Try to get the right spot within this zone, hold it and then move the direction of pressure on this spot in a small circle. You should aim to be on the most painful point. If repeated, this procedure should give a good appreciation of the depth needed. Follow all deep work with a more gentle generalised shoulder massage. The area where you did the deep work may still be tender but do not avoid it. This will help to dispel lactic acid and pain-inducing toxins from the area and stimulate the repair of the fascia.

a reminder of the muscles

the back

1 Trapezius

2 Levator scapulae

3 Rhomboids

4 Triceps

5 Latissimus dorsi

the front

1 Pectoral muscles

2 Subclavius muscles

3 Biceps

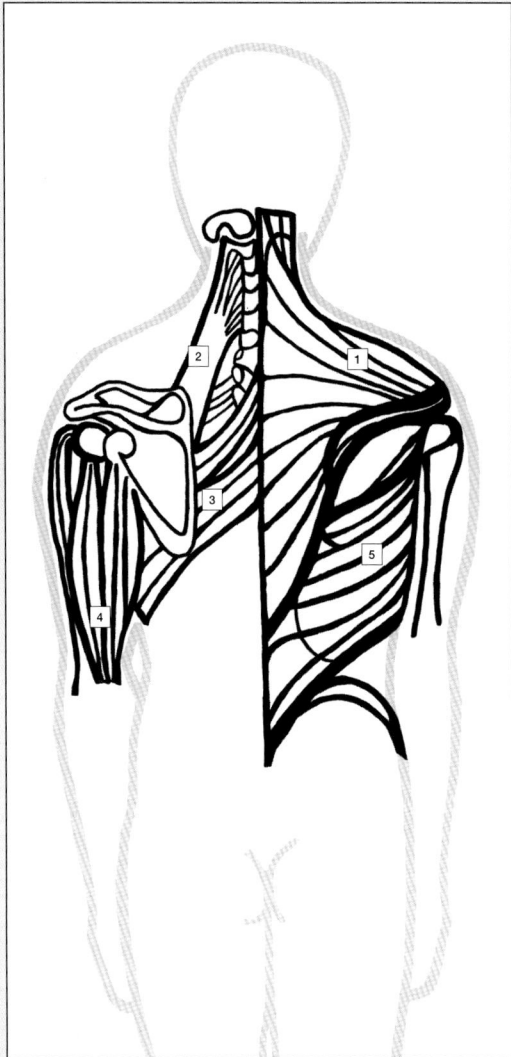
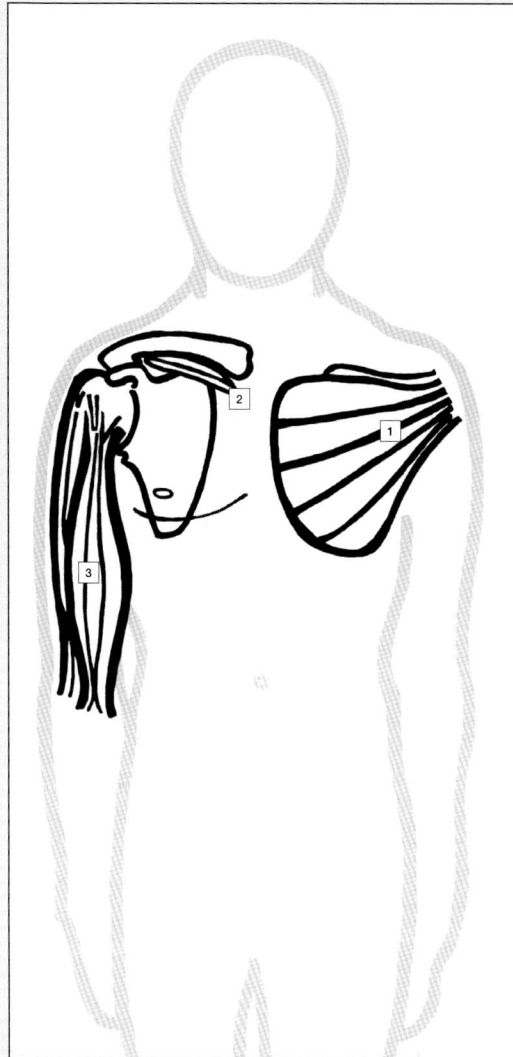

the side

1 Rotator cuff

2 Deltoid muscle

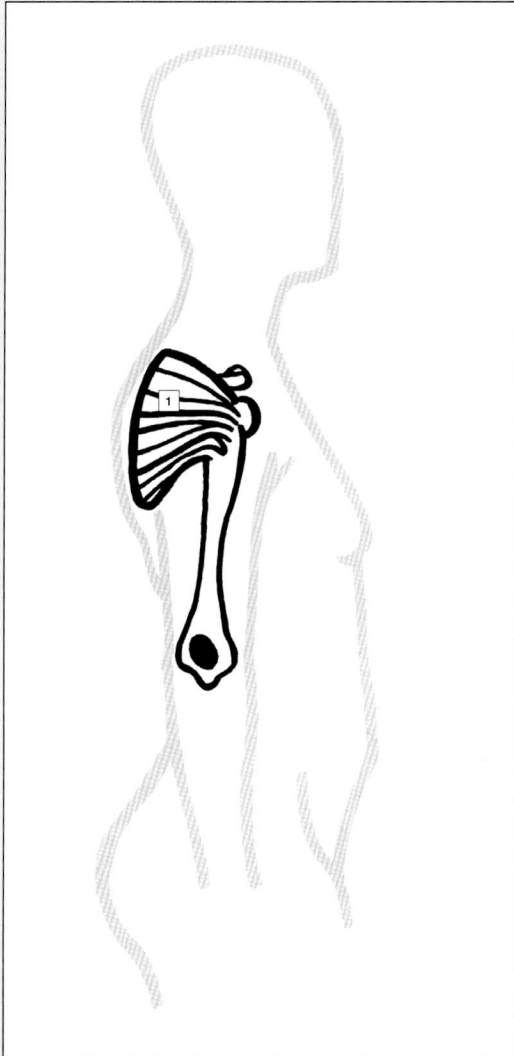

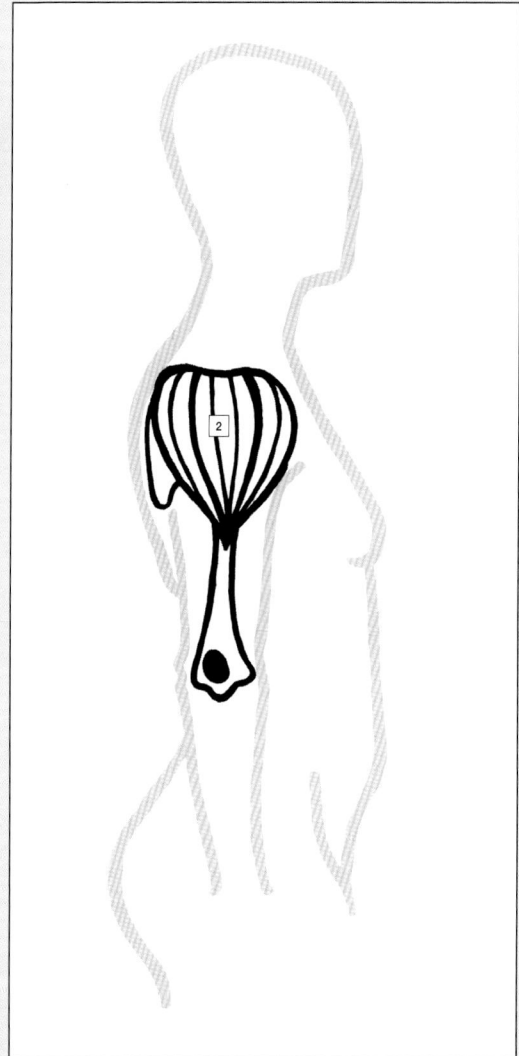

**frozen shoulder
anterior / posterior / lateral**

Follow steps 1–3 for the anterior, posterior and lateral diagnosis.

step 1

Here the pain is characterised by a sharp stinging in the front of the shoulder with even the most innocuous of activities. The pain may last for several minutes.

- Perform several deep slow strokes in one direction from the elbow towards the head only. You should feel a long tight band up the arm with nodules embedded in it.

- Moving upwards through the band, apply slow and steady pressure on these nodules.

- Follow this by a more gentle massage to the whole arm (upwards only).

PATIENT LYING ON THE GOOD SIDE
(or better side if bilateral)

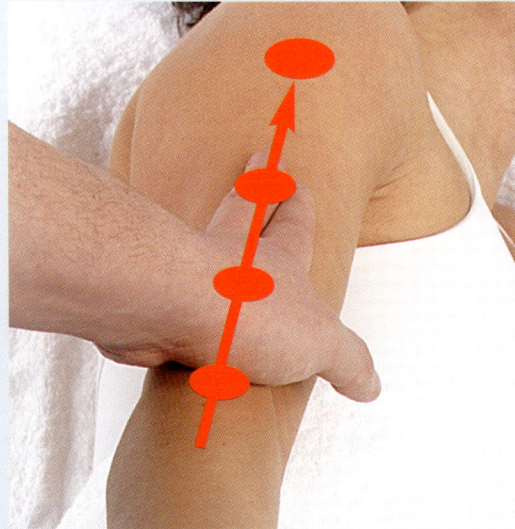

Direction stroke of pressure

IMPORTANT

Repeat steps 1–3 several times
for 2-4 minutes each. For all cases.

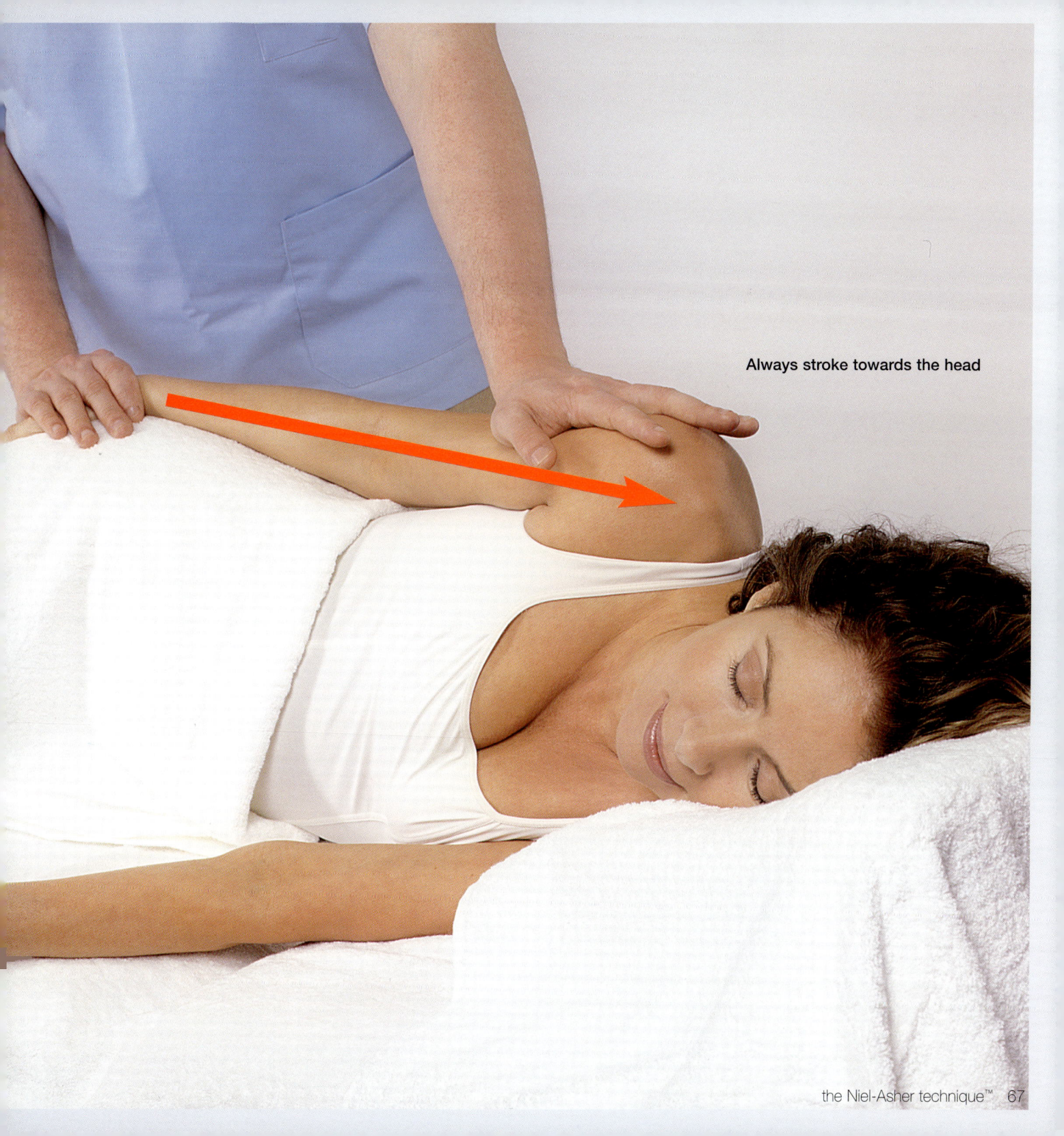

Always stroke towards the head

**frozen shoulder
anterior / posterior / lateral**

Follow steps 1–5 for the anterior, posterior and lateral diagnosis.

step 2

- Lying on the side, let the upper arm hang off the bed as much as possible.

- Now find the trigger point located in the joint capsule.

- Use deep sustained pressure on this point. Ask the patient to breathe in and out slowly and allow the hand and arm to get heavier and drop toward the floor with the breathing.

- Hold this point for up to 3 minutes, sometimes, if the pain eases quickly, you can change your direction of pressure within the nodule and hold this spot for a few minutes.

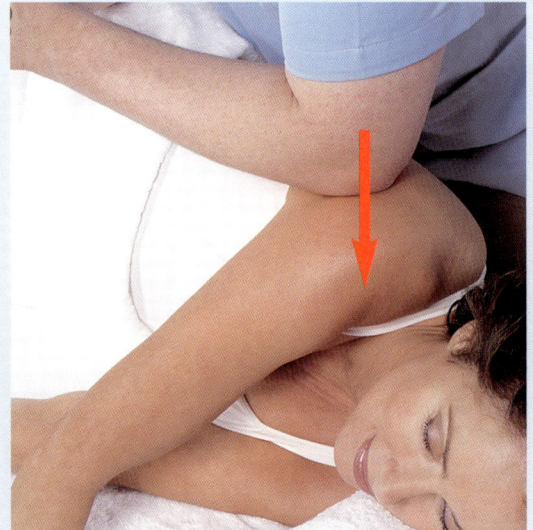

Lying on the side with arm dropped

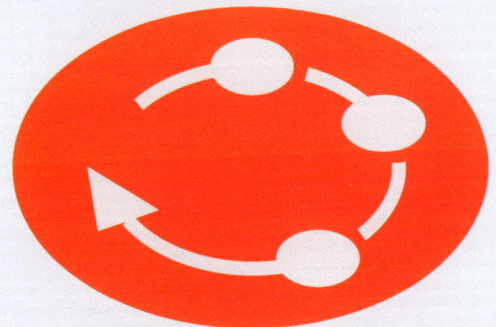

Direction of pressure within zone

Trigger points for stretching capsule

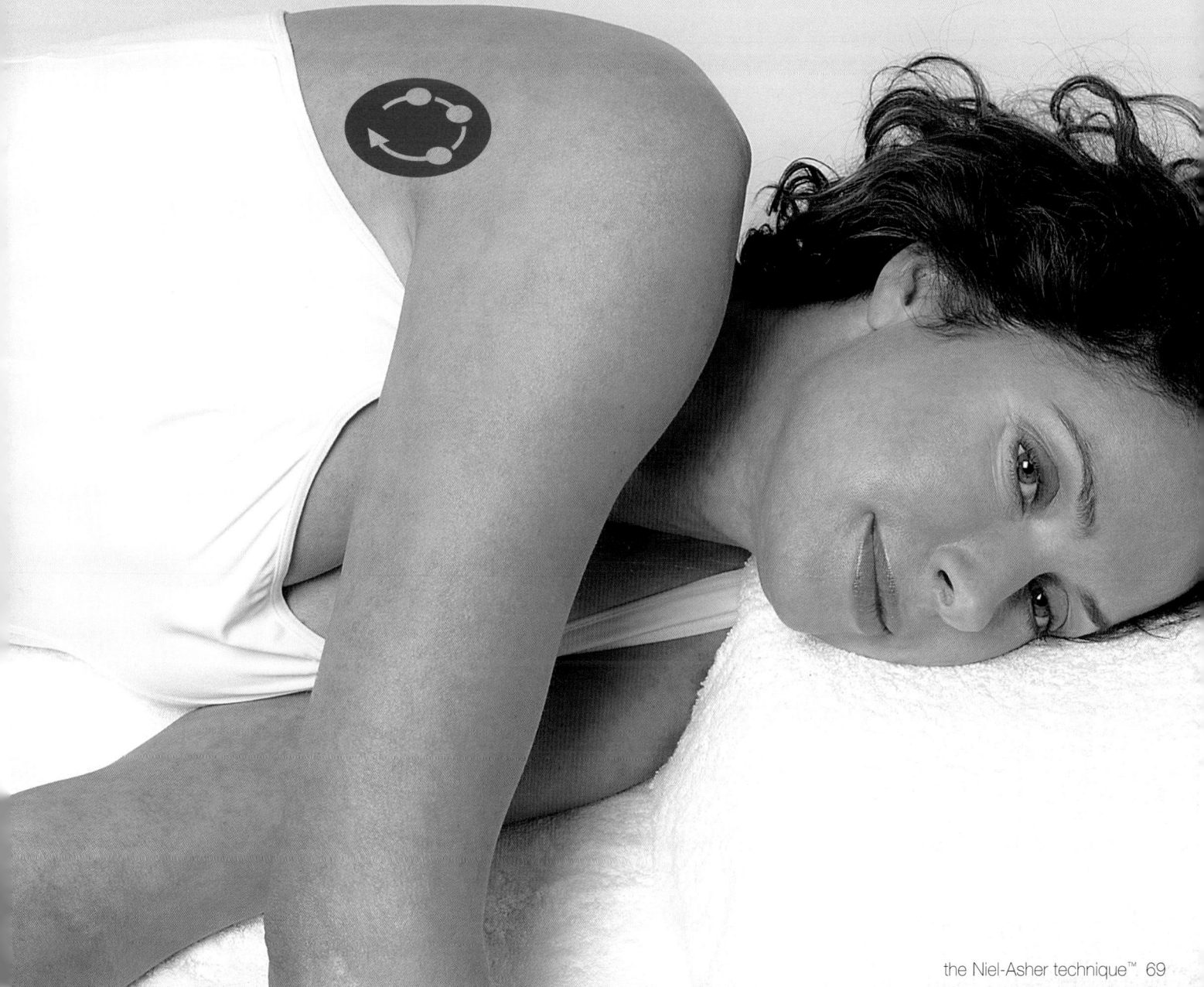

**frozen shoulder
anterior / posterior / lateral**

Follow steps 1–5 for the anterior, posterior and lateral diagnosis.

step 3

- Gently bring the arm back to the side; it may well be sore.

- Now you are going to move the bent arm in small circles, gradually increasing them to larger complete circles (circumduction).

- It is important that the patient's arm is completely heavy and relaxed and that the person performing the technique takes all the weight.

- Do not force the arm; take it to the pain zone and then come away about 20%. Use slow, confident movements.

- Do this several times.

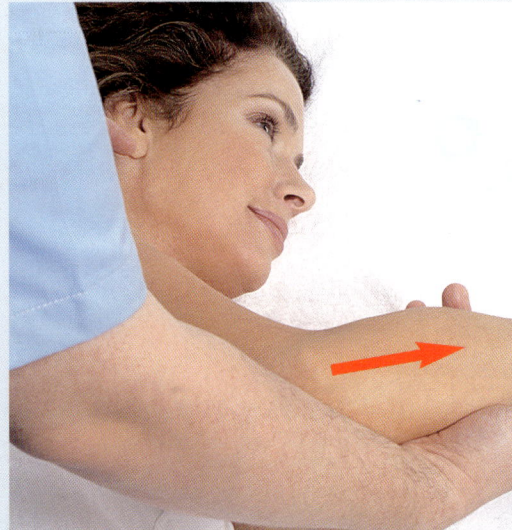

Beginning of circle

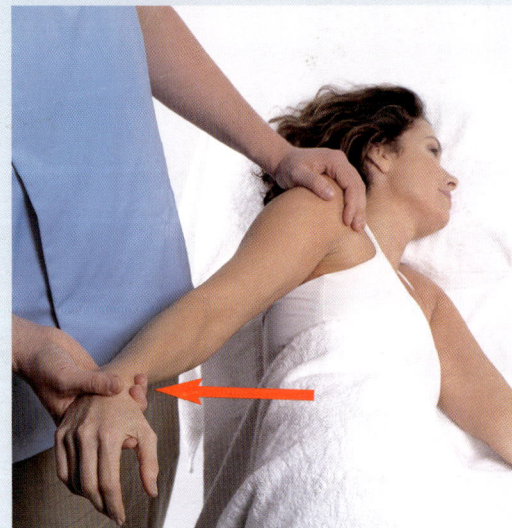

You can also take the arm backwards

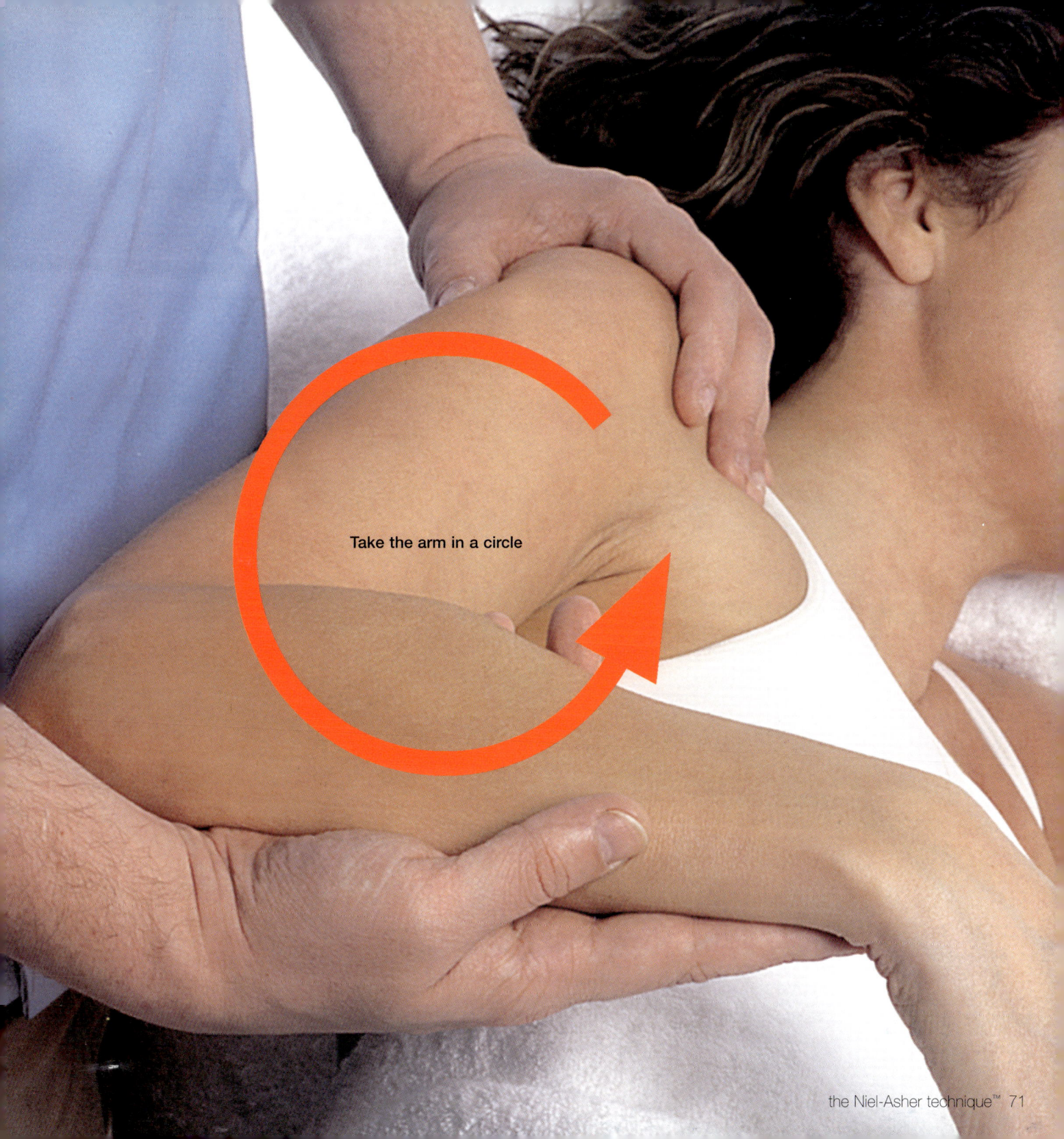

Take the arm in a circle

anterior step 4

This is a direct technique.

- With the patient on their back work slowly up the biceps tendon. Move towards the head only.

- Pause on the nodules along the tendon; these are fascial tetherings and may be inflamed.

- As you approach the shoulder, you should feel a particularly tender trigger point near the shoulder. This is where the biceps tendon joins the capsule; I often find the fascia to be particularly thickened at this point.

- Hold the trigger point for up to 3 minutes until it is completely pain free.

- Do not come away early as this may trigger a spasm. I use my elbow for comfort, but you can use your thumbs if you like - but go slowly and carefully.

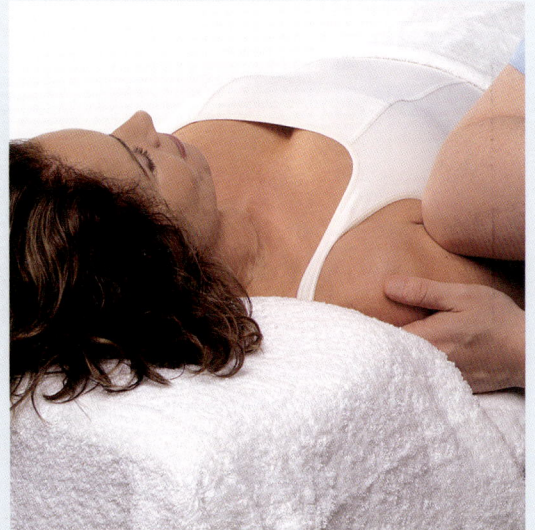

Move up the biceps tendon

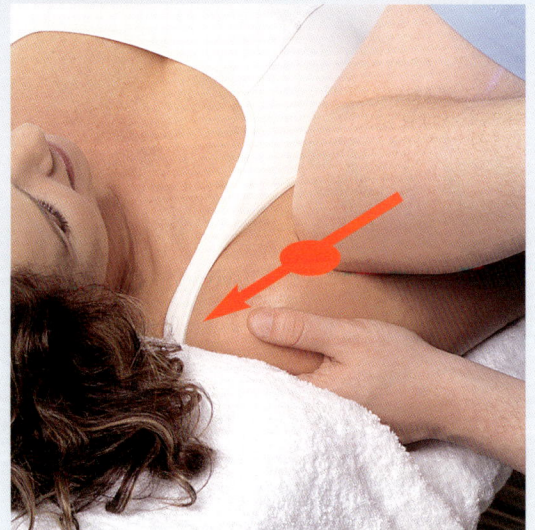

Holding at the trigger point

frozen shoulder
anterior / posterior / lateral

Follow steps 1–5 for the anterior, posterior and lateral diagnosis.

anterior step 5

This is an indirect technique.

- Turn the patient onto their back. Now using the middle fingers of your hand press deeply on the trigger point in the hot zone in the middle of the shoulder blade (infraspinatus).

- Use deep sustained pressure on this point. This can be extremely painful so ease into it, move clockwise around the zone until the pressure on this point can be felt 'inside' the shoulder joint.

- Hold this for a while with sustained pressure until this point relaxes and is no longer painful. This can take a while.

- If you get the right spot, the patient should feel referred pain in the front of the shoulder (biceps area).

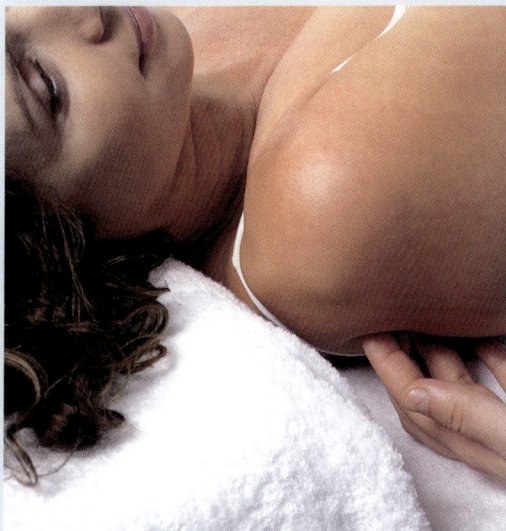

Position of trigger point

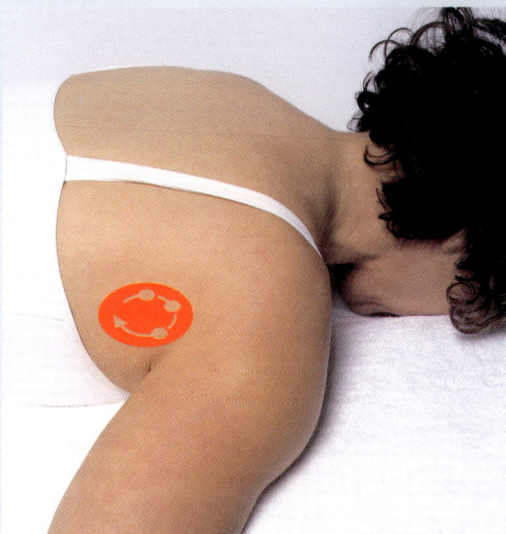

As seen from the back

combinations and modifications

About 20% of the cases I see involve a combination of anterior, posterior and lateral adhesions. In these cases a combination of all the above treatments may be appropriate.

• You can put a rolled up towel under the patient's arm when the patient is on their side. This acts as a fulcrum when you massage up the outer arm and stretches the joint capsule.

• Sometimes pulling the arm straight (traction) when the patient is lying on their side may be useful.

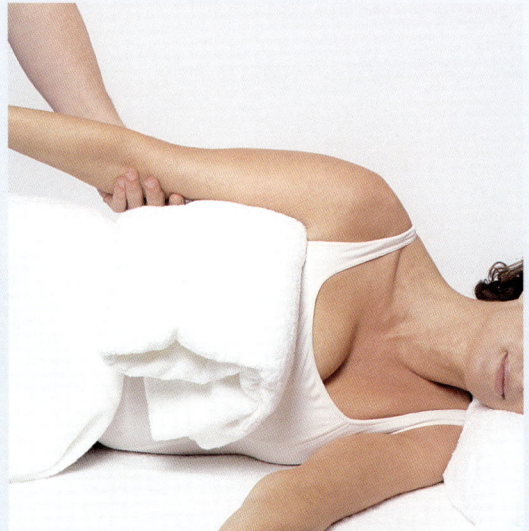

Towel as a fulcrum with traction

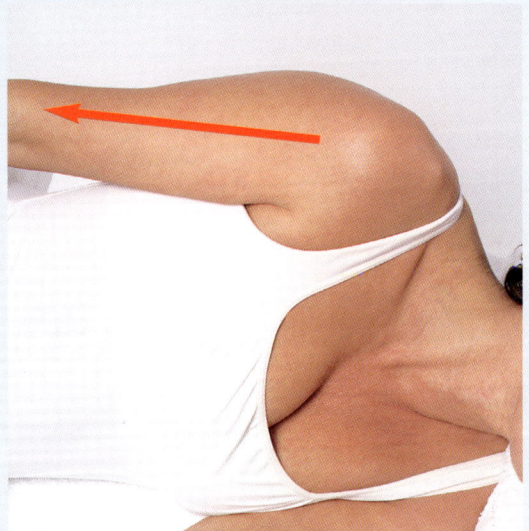

Traction with support

NOTES

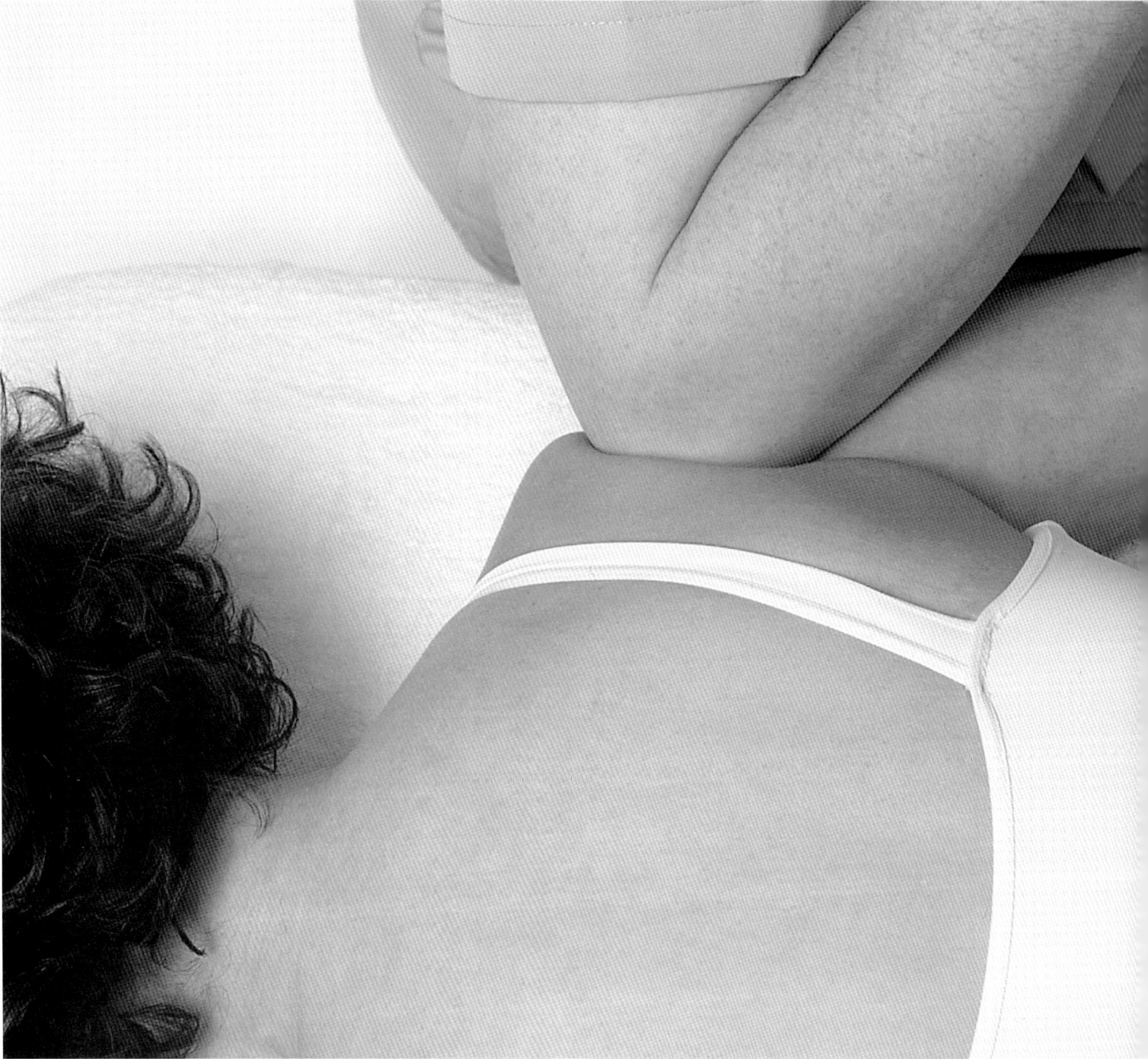

During the initial painful phase, rest may be useful as this gives inflamed tissue a chance to heal. Rest, however, does not mean using a sling; this is only appropriate in rare cases, after a fracture or surgery. Prolonged immobilisation has been demonstrated to aggravate the symptoms; in fact, it may even precipitate a frozen shoulder. Instead, try a combination of rest and some of the gentle exercises below. The use of non-steroidal anti-inflammatory medication (NSAIDs) has also proved useful in reducing tissue inflammation, because it inhibits the formation of various inflammatory substances. In some people this type of medication may cause stomach or skin problems, so please consult your doctor first. More gentle options include homeopathic arnica, ruta gravis and rhus tox. Some herbal medications have also proved effective in reducing inflammation. Rest is not so important in the frozen and thawing phases of a frozen shoulder (you have probably rested enough).

sleeping position

Night pain and sleeplessness are possibly the worst aspects of having a frozen shoulder, especially in the early days. At first, you probably will not be able to tolerate pressure on your affected side. As your symptoms ease, however, you will find you can gradually ease into some type of position. The degree of night pain is directly proportionate to the amount of inflammation within the joint.

Some comfort, if not relief, can be obtained by:

• Lying on your back with a pillow lengthways under the affected arm(s) and shoulders, supporting them.
• Lying on the good side with a pillow or towel over your waist and under the arm.

ice

Ice can be particularly beneficial, especially in the acute first and second phases when the inflammation is most active. You may feel sceptical about this, but so many people have enthusiastically described the relief they felt from applying ice to their shoulders that it's certainly worth trying.

• Wrap some crushed ice or frozen peas in a damp towel and place over the front of the shoulder joint. Leave it there for five to ten minutes.
• Let the area rest without ice for five to ten minutes and repeat.

You can also apply the ice to the back of the shoulder joint, the top, the side or other areas where there is acute pain. This is especially true in a posterior capsulitis. It is a good idea to ice the front of the shoulder even if it is not painful.

The ice regimen should be repeated as often as possible. When ice is not available or appropriate (at work, cinema etc) then cold sprays or gels can be useful – ask your pharmacist about them.

NB: never apply ice directly to the skin as it burns and leaves brown marks.

heat

In the early stages of a frozen shoulder, the direct application of heat is not a good idea, though a warm bath can be helpful.

Warm packs / hot water bottles that are not too hot can be applied in the second and third phases.

If you have found that heat does give you relief, then an alternating cycle of ice/warm/ice can be tried.

posture

- Try not to sleep with your arms above your head. This inhibits shoulder tissue repair, which occurs mainly at night.
- Avoid carrying heavy bags or cases for long distances; this has been demonstrated to precipitate tears in the supraspinatus muscle, a vital shoulder muscle.
- If you work standing up all day, take regular breaks where you can sit and rest the arms on a chair; the weight of the arms hanging has been demonstrated to cut off the blood supply to major shoulder muscles.
- If you are driving all day, or keeping your arms in a fixed position, take a regular break; this is because the muscles become fatigued and lactic acid builds up in the muscles, which over time can cause serious damage.
- If you work in front of a computer typing, take regular breaks. This is a law in many countries because of eyestrain but the effect on the shoulders is as in the point above.
- Be aware of your posture; the shoulder girdle operates best when the shoulders are held back and in correct alignment. 'Round shoulders' and long-term poor posture causes the shoulder muscles and joints to work inefficiently and can lead to 'pinching' of the tissues as the arms are used, causing further damage.

One of the protective postures that people with frozen shoulder adopt is to hunch the affected shoulder forwards, bend the arm at the elbow, and cradle the arm to the body. It is very important to avoid the sling position, which only compounds the problem. In this position the biceps muscle is contracted; stressing the tendon and eventually causing shortening. The best thing to do is straighten your arm and allow it to hang by the side of the body. Initially you should use the affected arm as little as possible, but as your pain diminishes you can swing the arm in walking.

re-positioning the shoulders

The following exercise may be useful in re-setting the shoulder posture. Ideally you should do it every day; failing that, try to aim for every other day. It can be uncomfortable at first, but should not be unbearable. If you cannot lie on the floor without severe pain then wait a week or so and then try again.

- Place a duvet or thick towel on the floor and lie on it, face up.
- Place pillows under both elbows and forearms.
- Rest your hands on your stomach, palms down. If that's not possible just rest them on the pillows.
- Stay in this position for 20 minutes. Listen to the radio if you like.

Very slowly the shortened tissues at the back of the shoulder should stretch. This allows the hands to drop towards the chest. The tight muscles at the front of the chest will also relax, allowing the shoulders to 'sink back'.

when acute spasm strikes

A sudden movement, such as reaching for a falling cup, holding a door that is suddenly blown open or even being bumped into on the street, can cause a sudden increase in painful muscle spasms. These acute attacks

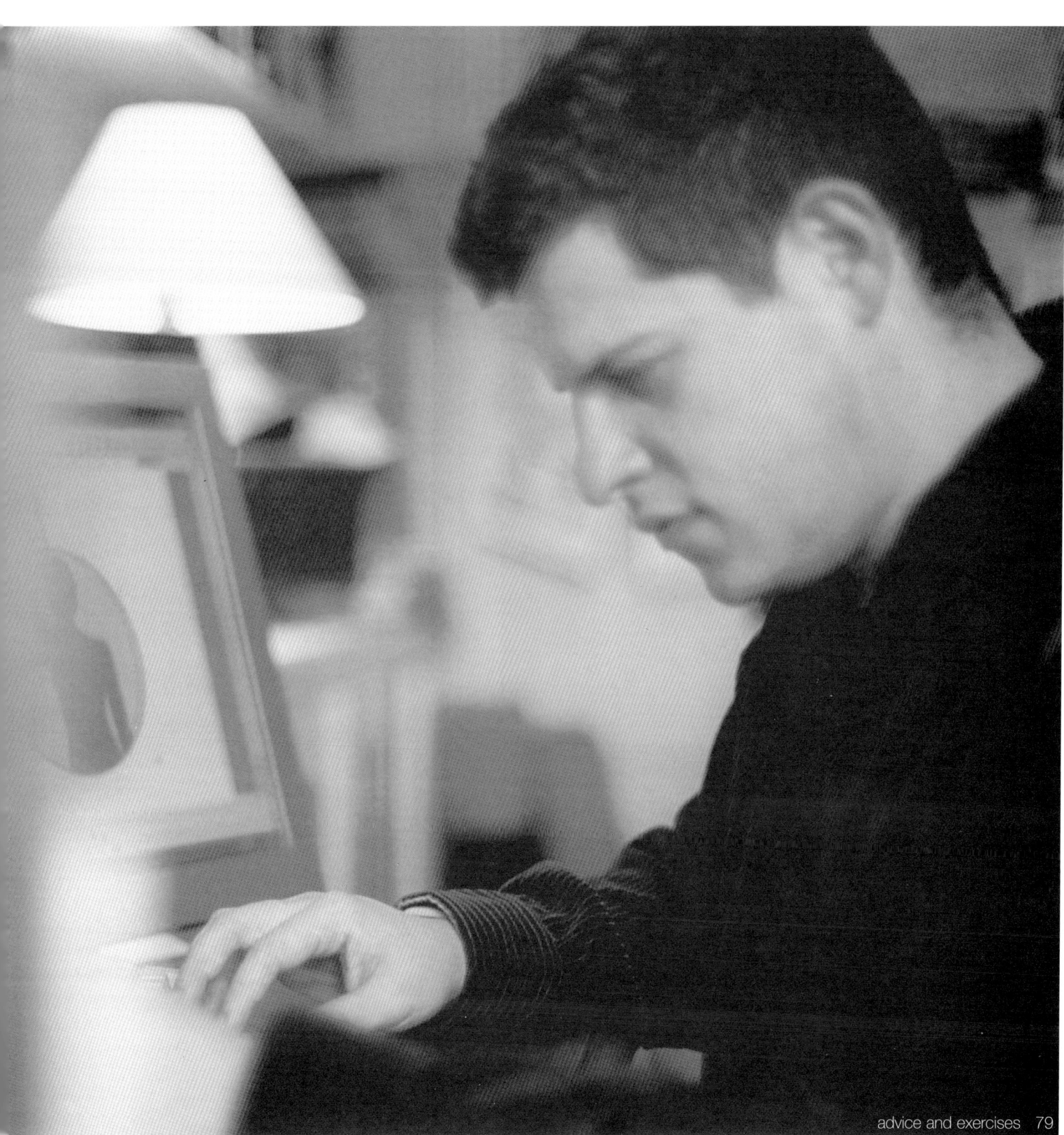

of severe pain can add anxiety to the sufferer's already considerable burden. Most patients find that they can stop these attacks by doing the exercise below. First this phenomenon needs to be understood.

The acute pain is caused when the thickened biceps tendon (long head) slips in its shallow specialised groove. This is because the biceps tendon sheath is thickened from inflammation.

When an unexpected movement goes through the joint, the muscles all lock into protective spasm. Going into the spasm by flexing the arm can reverse this sudden pain. The muscles no longer 'see' a need for their activity and it is switched off. However, there is quite a fine line between gently going with the muscles and creating a further 'challenge', so remember that the exercise described below is subtle and should be performed slowly and gently.

- Rest the hand on a table or chair back with the palm down.
- Allow the weight of the arm to rest on the hand, causing slight compression at the shoulder joint. Breath deeply and slowly. It helps to apply the pressure as you breath out.
- It is as though you were about to lean your body weight on your hand, while only applying a fraction of the force.

daily life

As mentioned above, the best position for the arm during the initial stages of the condition is to let the straightened arm hang loosely at your side, but that is not to say that you should let the frozen shoulder interfere too much with your daily life. In the face of constant pain, sleep deprivation and decreased joint mobility it is very hard to feel life is normal. One of the really unpleasant aspects of having a frozen shoulder is the sense of isolation that the above symptoms frequently cause. 'My shoulder really hurts' doesn't come close to describing the ordeal. It is very hard indeed for people to understand what you are going through. Such circumstances can lead to a sense of vulnerability and depression. In order to combat this, it is vital to stay as fully engaged with your life as possible. Be patient with your loved ones when they pester you with constant enquiries about your shoulder. Some will expect more of you than you are able to give. Others 'leave you in peace' just when you would like some sympathy. Most people are not good at dealing with the pain of others, especially someone they love. Be sure to set out very clearly what can and can't be expected of you at work.

impediments to progress

Try to watch out for bad habits that contribute to the severity of your symptoms. These are often unconscious and include making repeated circular movements with the elbow, forcing the arm into an uncomfortable stretch, tensing the elbow against the side of the body, leaning your elbows on your desk, holding the arm in the sling position, not drinking enough water, carrying a heavy bag on one shoulder and tensing into the discomfort. When pain strikes, it is vital that you take a deep breath and let the muscles relax as you breath out.

the light at the end of the tunnel

Patients usually feel a good enough improvement at the end of their first session to give them hope. However, the initial improvement is usually short-lived - from a few hours to a couple of days. You may also notice a slight aggravation of your symptoms; these are the after-effects of the treatment itself. It is perfectly normal to feel a bit battered; so do not worry.

The benefits should last a little longer after each session. However, no two patients are quite the same.

This treatment will accelerate you through the condition, not stop it in its tracks. If you are starting from the beginning the first phase, you may get a bit less movement or a bit more pain initially. Sometimes the the first movement in one particular direction is slow to respond, or that the night pain continues even when people are relatively pain-free during the day. Some regain lost movement quickly but still experience pain. Others are pain-free after only a short time, but continue to grapple with the disability of limited movement. There can also be a 'plateau' when little change seems to occur. In my experience all patients will end up the same – with little to no pain and a functional if not full range of movement. Of those few patients who we have failed to cure completely, a good percentage report sufficient improvement to enable them to live more normal lives. Don't lose heart.

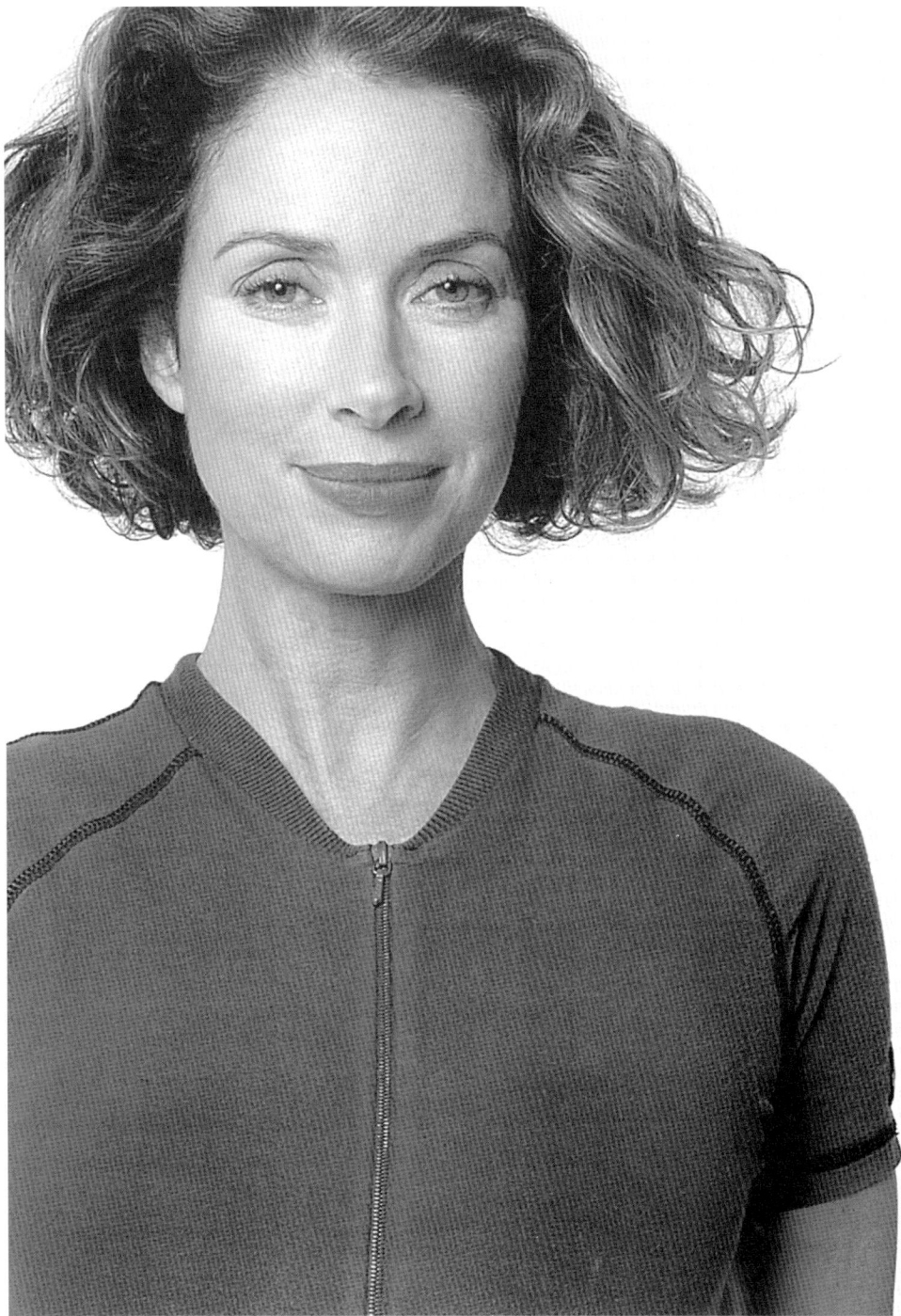

exercises

There are two aspects to exercise. First there is stretching and second there is strengthening.

In my experience, the timing at which to start exercising is very important. I will suggest some exercises that I have found useful for my own patients.

phase 1 – freezing

This is a crucial time for starting a gentle stretching regime. Gentle is the operative word. Your shoulder is likely to be very inflamed at the beginning of this phase but gently stretching the capsule three times per day for five minutes stops the adhesions getting too tight. If you are in too much pain, do as much as you can or stop completely for a few days. Remember to use ice for pain relief.

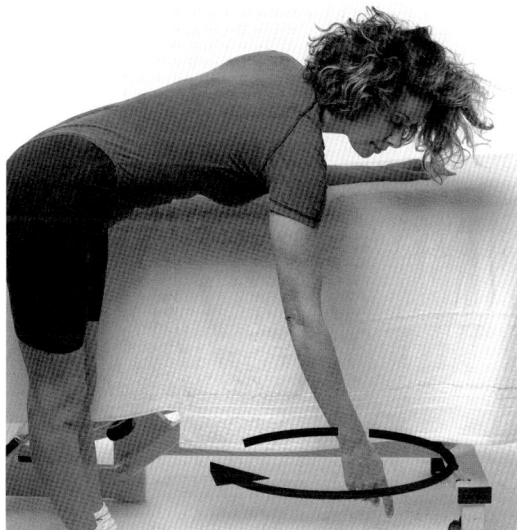

capsule stretching

This important exercise is best done gently in between each treatment session. Start with this passive exercise before you add any weights. It is very simple but easy to get wrong so please follow the instructions carefully.

- Bend forward at the waist
- Let the bad arm drop towards the floor under its own weight
- Feel the sense of tugging and traction in the shoulder joint
- You can support your other hand on a chair
- Move your body to make the hanging arm swing gently
- Use this method to swing or rock the arm in small to medium-sized circles

You may want to use ice (see page 85) after these sessions.

Shoulder shrugging can be performed five times daily for 2 – 5 minutes. You can move both shoulders at the same time and then independently. Raise the shoulder up to the neck and push them downwards towards the floor. Be careful if you have a neck problem. You can then gently rotate the shoulders in circles together then independently, again, take it nice and slow if you have any neck problems.

shoulder shrugging

- Stand upright
- Shrug your shoulders upwards as high as you can for 8 seconds
- Let the shoulders drop
- Squeeze the shoulders downwards
- Repeat 3 times

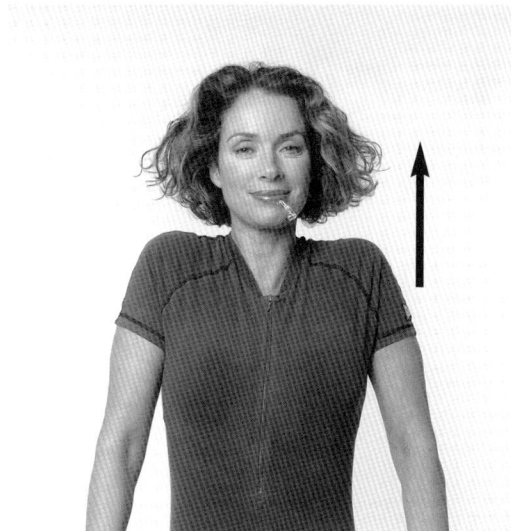

shoulder rotation

- Stand upright
- Keep the hands by the sides
- Rotate the shoulder in a circle
- Change direction
- Repeat on other arm
- Repeat slowly for 2 minutes

You will know you are approaching the end of the first phase when your night pain reduces significantly. This indicates that there is less inflammation and less 'internal' burning inflammation. Now is the time to start 'stepping-up' your exercise programme by adding slightly deeper stretches of the capsule and weights where indicated.

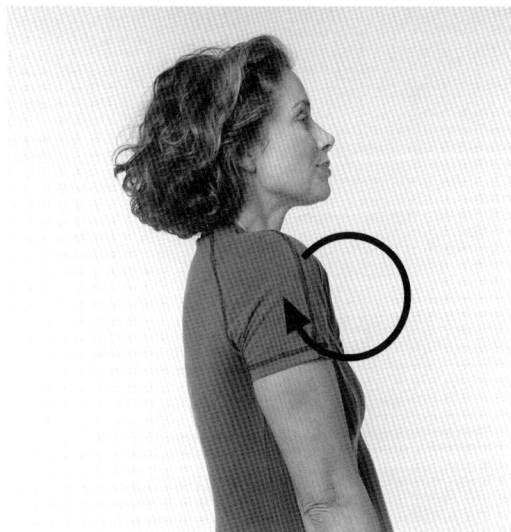

Shoulder shrugging

Shoulder rotation

phase 2 – frozen

Keep going with the phase I exercises. You can now use a small weight to improve your capsular stretch and add some strength to the shoulder muscles.

You can also add the following exercises:

crawl the wall
part 1

- Turn sideways to the wall
- Using the bad arm, gently crawl the fingers up the wall
- Remember where you get to
- Crawl back down the wall
- Repeat several times

part 2

- Turn to face the wall and repeat the exercise

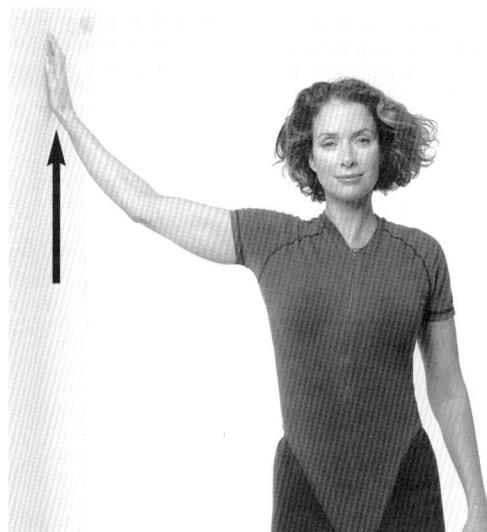

Crawl the wall - part 1

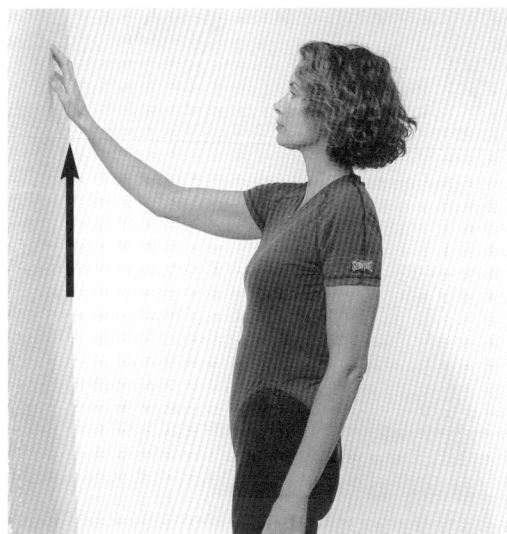

part 2

simple shoulder stretches

- These are simple exercises that can be performed sitting at a dining table.

front of shoulder

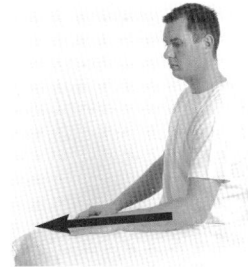

- Sit square to a table and lean forwards on a bent elbow.

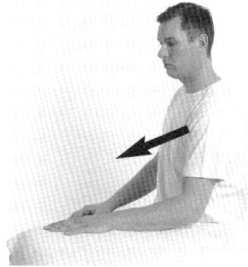

stretching the back of the shoulder

- Sitting at table crawl the hand forward and lean on it slightly until you feel a stretch at the back of the shoulder joint.

1. Front shoulder   **2. Back shoulder**

traction and stretch

- Sit on a table or plinth near to the edge
- Hold the table edge with the hand
- Gently lean away from the table edge
- You should feel a stretching in the shoulder and neck

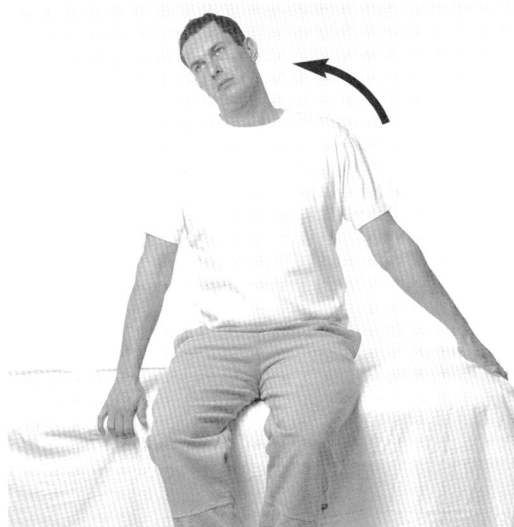

Traction and stretch

phase 3 – thawing

After a few weeks of performing the Niel-Asher technique™ and with the above stretches you should feel ready to strengthen your weak shoulder muscles. Remember they haven't been used properly for months, so take it gently. In my experience, 60% of people re-develop their muscle power just by going back to the normal every day activities. This is preferable. 40% of cases, however, really seem to need a bit of extra help. I have found adding the following exercises (to those already mentioned) useful in such circumstances,

strengthening

The following exercises involve either a using a small 1kg weight or using an elasticated resistance band. These should only be performed when the night pain has diminished more than 90%.

stretching using a 1kg weight

Lie on front using a small weight
- Lift the weight up and down slowly in a controlled manner. Then let it hang to the floor to pull on the shoulder joint.

- Swing the arm in circles slowly using the 1kg weight as in capsular stretching exercise.

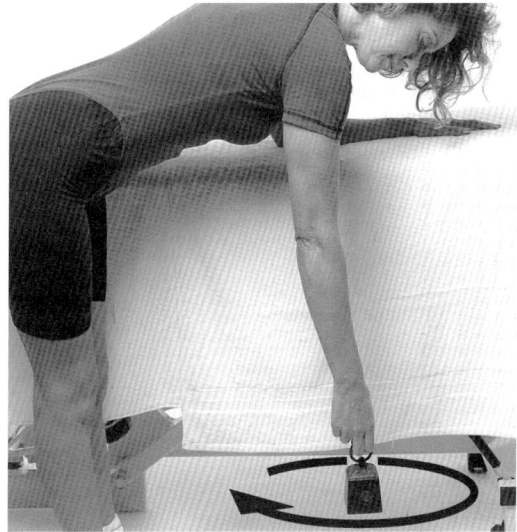

Using a 1kg weight

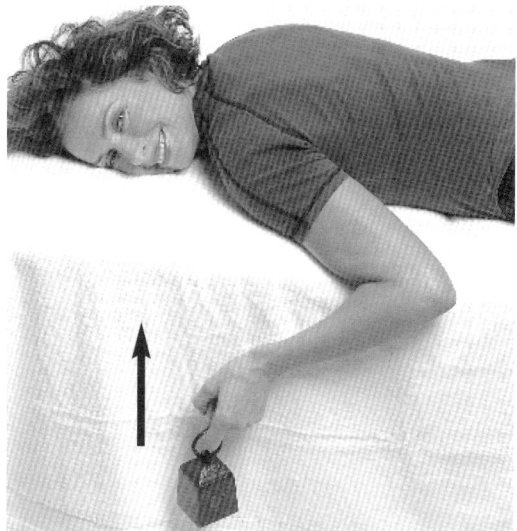

Using a small weight

elastic resistance rep-band™

This is a high quality latex-free product. It is a more advanced product than many cheaper alternatives.The way you hold the band is up to you but try varying your handhold every 3 days.

using an elastic resistance rep-band™

- 1. Starting at waist level, slowly pull both sides of the resistance band
- 2. Repeat half way up the chest
- 3. Repeat as high up as possible
- Repeat 1–8 times
- Be careful not to let it snap back
- Be controlled both on pulling and on relaxing
- You may want to build up to this
- If in pain, stop

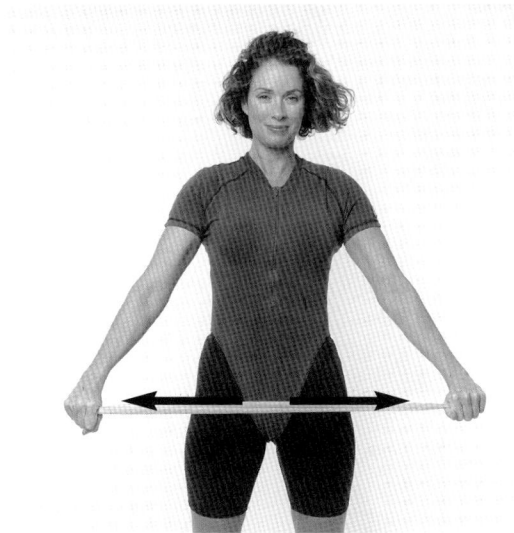

1

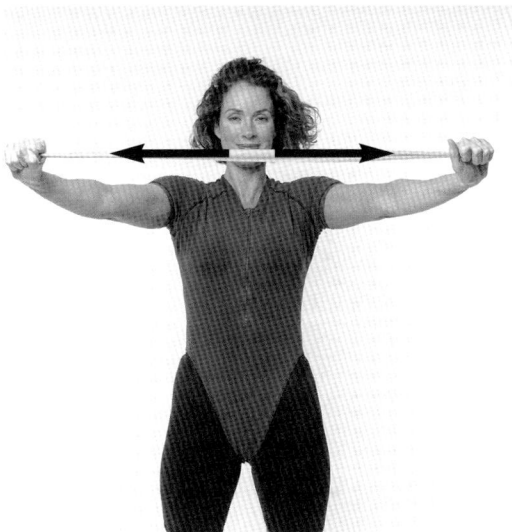

2

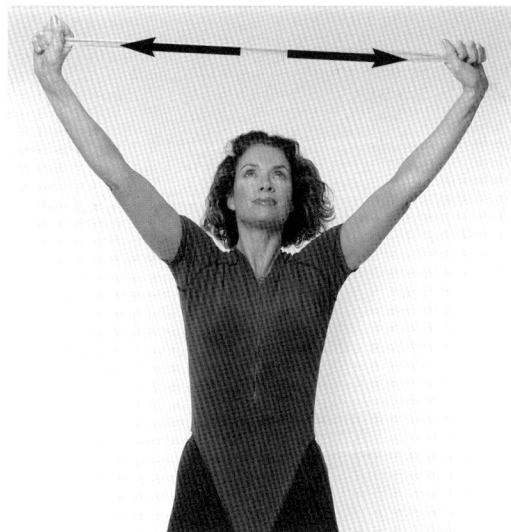

3

- Tie the band to a closed door handle
- Facing the door pull the band backwards with a straight arm
- Keep a slow and steady pressure

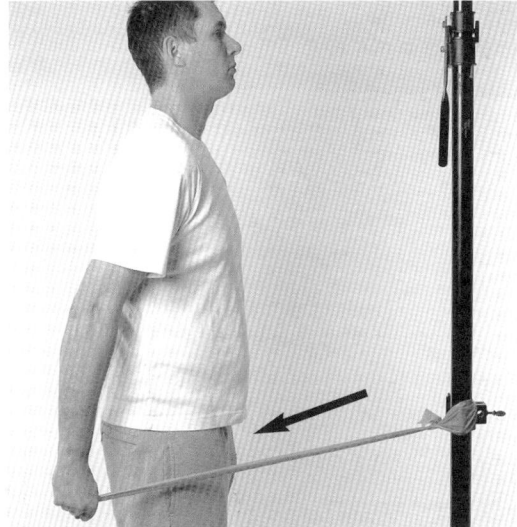

Band tied to a door handle

- Perform this exercise by pulling the band apart behind the back
- A towel may be used instead
- Go slowly
- Repeat 1–8 times
- Change arms

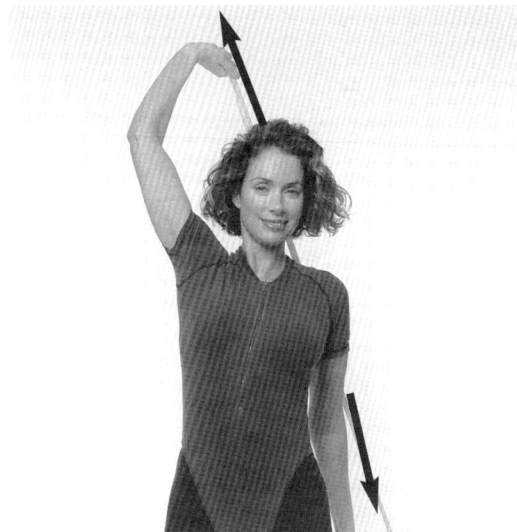

Band across the back

swimming

This is the main exercise I recommend to my patients. It is only advised in the second and third phases, once the night pain has gone. Do not swim for more than an hour with regular breaks every other lap. Any stroke you can manage will suffice initially. As you get more confident, you can experiment with the style. Expect the shoulder to ache initially; this will improve with time. Remember, your shoulder muscles will be very weak if you have not used them for many months. Do not overdo it; it is better to build things up slowly. Swimming has many benefits, most of which are well documented. The main benefits for rehabilitating a frozen shoulder are that the body-weight is reduced and that the water offers just the right amount of resistance, when swimming, to build up wasted muscles.

treatment reactions/side effects

We are used to going to the doctor and receiving a pill or remedy, which usually works within a few hours. However it has been demonstrated that the majority of people (70%) have a reaction to treatment after an osteopathic session. Treatment reactions are a natural part of the overall effect of osteopathy.

This is because osteopathy taps into the body's own healing mechanisms and these often take a few days to adjust and re-balance. Curiously, from the research it seemed that the worse the treatment reaction the better the improvement seems to be, (JACAM April 1997, June 1997).

some common treatment reactions / side effects

Tiredness, headaches, changes in bowel movement (diarrhoea or constipation), increased urinary frequency, joint aching (flu-like) and/or increased pain for about 24-48 hours. All the above seem worse for neck pain. Some people also feel emotional, vulnerable and/or tearful.

Drink plenty of water after treatment and rest when possible.

a treatment reaction commonly lasts for 2 – 3 days

If you feel worse after 2-3 days, please stop the treatment until the symptoms have settled. I have never seen a case get worse overall from my method. The only times people appear to feel worse is if they are in the freezing phase and their tissues are in exquisite pain / tenderness. Any treatment of tissues in this state will cause increased pain. If you are in this phase of the condition, it is advisable to let your symptoms settle for a few weeks and then try the method again.

finally

Thank you all so much for purchasing this programme. With your book, and dvd to reinforce it, you can start the process of getting better. I am very excited to be sharing my success with you all. As this technique is still new, you may find it difficult to find a properly trained practitioner. For more information on a practitioner near you visit www.frozenshoulder.com. If this programme works for you, please tell your friends or therapists about it. We are planning to run seminars in the Niel-Asher technique™ very soon. For maximum benefit you may wish to see a qualified practitioner in the Niel-Asher technique™. Information for practitioners will be updated on the website.

Best of luck

simeon

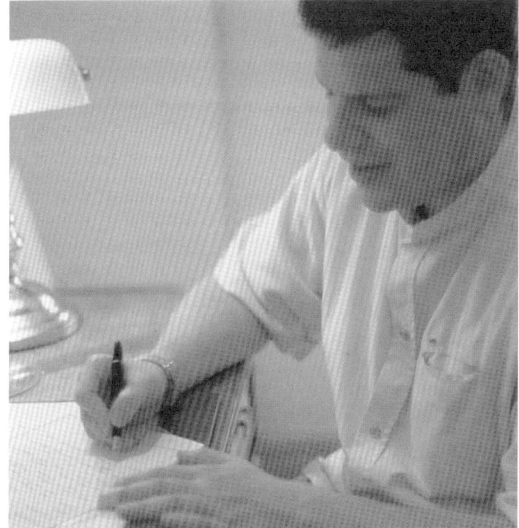

appendix

medical terms explained

acromion	Tip of shoulder - part of the shoulder blade
anterior	To the front - forward
arthritis	Wear and tear of joint cartilage and bone
arthrography	Operation involving the injection of dye into the shoulder joint
arthroscopy	Operation: keyhole surgery into a joint
avascular-necrosis	Loss of blood to a bone causing it to shrink and decay
Beçets syndrome	Medical condition in males related to NSU which can cause joint pain
biceps rupture	Complete tear of one of the biceps tendons
biceps tendonitis	Inflammation of the biceps tendons or tendon sheaths
bony spur	Excess formation of bone in the shape of a spur
cervical bar	Excess bone formation in the neck – often related to ageing
cervical myelopathy	Pressure on a nerve exiting the neck bones
cervical spine	Neck – top seven spinal vertebrae
cholelithiasis	Small stones that form in the gall bladder
cholycystitis	Inflammation of the gall bladder
circulatory	Relating to the blood vessels
clavicle	Collar-bone
collagen	Fibrous tissue, found throughout the body
congenital	Medical conditions which are present at birth
CT scans	Imaging technique using computerised tomography
degenerative	Wear and tear
degenerative arthritis	Wear and tear of joints – can be systemic or local
disc degeneration	Damage or wear to a spinal disc (jelly-filled)
dislocation	When a joint is displaced, often due to force
displaced fracture	Break in a bone which has not been re-set
functional	Related to the function
gastric ulcer	Inflamed erosion of stomach wall
gastrointestinal	Relating to the bowels
giant cell arteritis (GCA)	A condition related to polymyalgia rheumatica characterised by a sharp linear pain from the forehead to above the eye
genitourinary	Relating to the genital and urinary systems
goniometer	Instrument/ruler used to measure movement
gouty arthritis	A bad type of arthritis which results from gout
haematopoietic	Body systems involved in blood production
haemophiliac bleed	A bleed into a joint – more common in haemophiliacs

heart attack	Myocardial Infarction
humerus	Upper arm bone
hypercalcinosis	Increased production of calcium
hyperparathyroidism	Overproduction of parathyroid hormone which regulates bone deposition and remodelling
impingement	Trapped
infective	From an infection
labrum	Lip or cup (made of cartilage)
lateral	To the side
manipulation under anaesthesia (MUA)	Operation involving manipulation of the shoulder joint whilst under general anaesthetic
metabolic	Relating to the metabolism
metastasis	Secondary spread of cancer
monostotic	Relating to a single joint
MRI scans	Magnetic resonant imaging scans
myeloma	Disease of the lymph
neoplastic	Cancerous or new growth
nerve root	Where the nerve starts
nerve root compression	Compression of a nerve near its root
neurological	Relating to the nerves
non-specific urethritis (NSU)	Condition involving an infection of the urethra often caused by sexual intercourse
NSAIDs	Non-steroidal anti-inflammatory medication
orthopedic	Branch of medicine specialising in bone/joint pain
osteochondromatosis	Cancer of a bone – very rare
osteomalacia	Malformation of bone due to lack of nutrition
osteopaenia	Malformation of bone
osteophytic	Outgrowth of bone
osteoporosis	Ageing condition of bone which makes it brittle
osteosarcoma	Rare bone tumour
Paget's disease	Ageing disease where bone does not solidify properly and becomes bendy; often occurs in skull bones
Pancoast tumour	Lung tumour at top of lung
Parkinson's disease	Progressive wasting disease of the nervous system
polymyalgia	Disease of elderly especially females characterised
rheumatica	By tenderness of shoulder or pelvic girdle, fever +/- GCA
posterior	To the back
prolapse	Collapse or squashing
prostate	Gland above bladder in men which swells/ hardens with age
pseudo-gout	Gout-like symptoms but non-uric crystals

radioisotope scans	Scan of bones using radioactive salts
Raynaud's	Painful numbing bluish whiteness and coldness of hands or feet due to a change of nerve supply to blood vessels
Reiter's syndrome	Medical condition in males related to NSU which can cause joint pain and conjunctivitis
respiratory	Relating to heart and lungs
reticulo-endothelial	Relating to the system of collagen cells and skin
rheumatologist	Specialists in soft tissue pain
rotator cuff tear	Tear or damage to the rotator cuff tendon
septic arthritis	Arthritis secondary to infection
shoulder–hand	Rare manifestation of frozen shoulder syndrome
syndrome	Where pain is felt in the elbow, wrist and hand
spiral fracture	Spiral breakage of long bones common in shoulder-humerus
stomach cancer	Cancer of the stomach, which may not show up for years or may sometimes present as left shoulder pain
stroke	Brain damage often, one-sided, often caused by a blood clot
sub-acromial bursitis	Inflammation of fluid pad under the tip of the shoulder
thoracic outlet syndrome	Condition characterised by hand pain, throbbing or numbness, secondary to pressure on nerves/blood vessels
traumatic	Relating to a fall, car accident or trauma
x-rays	Medical investigation using radioactive radium

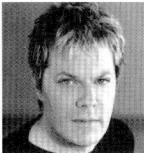